cassandra

chakra power

— for —
healing and harmony

quantum
LONDON • NEW YORK • TORONTO • SYDNEY

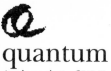

quantum

An imprint of W. Foulsham & Co. Ltd
The Publishing House, Bennetts Close,
Cippenham, Slough, Berkshire, SL1 5AP, England

ISBN 0–572–02749–4

Typeset by Grafica, Bournemouth, Dorset
Printed in Great Britain by St. Edmundsbury Press, Bury St. Edmunds, Suffolk

Contents

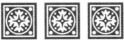

Introduction

Science acknowledges that the universe and all that is in it is composed of constantly changing particles of energy and not solid matter. Moreover, the system is interdependent, so that action in one part reverberates as reaction in others. The ancients of Africa, India, the Americas and Oceania knew this fact thousands of years ago.

Indeed, it is hypothesised that awareness of the chakras – the vortexes of psychic energy through which the life force is channelled in the human body, mind and spirit – came first out of Africa and reached India and the Far East with the early migration of tribes. In the Far East, the chakra tradition has long been central to philosophy and religion. Chakras under different names have been used as foci for empowerment and healing for thousands of years in many cultures.

Working with the seven main chakras that correspond to the colours of the rainbow, offers one of the simplest and yet most potent ways of regulating and integrating mind, body and soul. The chakras also control the flow of energies to and from the aura, the rainbow-coloured energy field surrounding the human body, as well as that of animals, plants and even crystals. The aura acts as a receiver and transmitter for influences from the cosmos, the Earth and those with whom we interact and is the first area to reflect the effects of these interactions upon health and harmony. A bright luminous rainbow aura indicates that the chakras are likewise operating at peak efficiency.

Picture a vast ocean of universal energy flowing in and out of our psychic channels, energising the physical and spirit bodies. Our personal vibrations are carried out into that vast sea, and so alter in a small but significant way the composition of the universe. Under the energy interchange system, good vibes really do make the world a happier place. In the same way, the accumulation of energies from people, animals, plants, places – and also angels, devas or higher nature essences, spirit guides and the wise ancestors who live in different dimensions – influence us as their knowledge flows through our chakras.

The importance of the chakras for well-being

When the chakras are open and functioning well, they receive energy and vitality from the universal life force and ensure that our interactions on every level are positive and enriching. At their most efficient, chakras are able to filter out any impurities or negativity, or transform them into impetus for change and progress. Indeed, at this optimum efficiency, all levels – physical, emotional, psychic and spiritual – are in harmony. In this state our bodies can resist illness by triggering the innate immune system, our minds think clearly and concentrate on vital issues, but we can also tap intuitively into the vast cosmic memory bank that is accessible in this ocean of energy. As Einstein stated, matter can neither be created nor destroyed – or as T.S. Eliot put it rather more elegantly in the *Four Quartets:* 'All time is eternally present.'

It is rare for all the chakras to be working flat out, and blockages in them can dam up energies or channel them into inappropriate reactions or ways of viewing the world, other people and ourselves. Chakra healing then, whether of a specific ailment, disease or a general disharmony not only corrects the problem but also enables the patient or ourselves, if we are working with our own chakras, to operate in the world in a more harmonious and effective way.

Chakras, however, are much more than a regulating system. They form a ladder, in the same way that the Jewish esoteric or Kabbalistic Tree of Life offers through its ten spheres (or *sephiroth*) both ascent from the material world to higher levels of awareness and the grounding of those higher energies in the everyday world of the individual seeker. For, unlike the followers of the Hindu and Buddhist traditions, many seekers of spirituality in the West do not want to escape from the everyday world, but to enrich it through developing their chakra power.

It is sometimes said that when we are born, we are incarnated into the lowest or Root chakra level of existence and functioning – the physical body – after moving steadily downwards from the highest plane of existence, which is identified with the Crown chakra through conception and growth in the womb. Then we rise again to the highest sphere of existence as we return to the realm of Spirit in death. People who believe in reincarnation see this as a continuing cycle until the point where the spirit is so evolved it no longer wishes or needs to become incarnate.

However, each of the seven main chakra levels of existence (see page 14) is of equal importance. The first and lowest major chakra, the Root chakra, is one that enables us to feel comfortable in our bodies and with ourselves and so is the firm foundation without which spiritual evolution is not possible. For many people, the seventh and highest level of existence that is linked with the Crown chakra becomes more important in old age, as we move closer to Spirit once more. Such a feeling may occur only occasionally, during events that the US psychologist Abraham Maslow called the peak experience – those moments out of time when we feel at one with the universe and with the source of divinity, however we envisage it.

The exploration and development of the powers inherent at each chakra level bring psychic and spiritual gifts, as well as improved relationships and interactions in our work. Although in Eastern traditions, yoga is an integral part of chakra work and I have suggested useful books on this discipline (see page 155), you can use a number of other methods that I will describe in subsequent chapters. These are just as potent and fit easily into everyday Western life. Yoga was developed in a very different world where long hours of meditation and bodywork formed an integral part of the day. Increasing numbers of people in the West are finding yoga helpful as part of their spiritual development, but others have found it physically and mentally problematic and have become discouraged from working with their chakras. Methods are just tools that offer one way of achieving a desired result and so in this book, as any other, you should select the ways that are right for you and discard the rest. If you do want to learn yoga, there are many classes and, initially, personal training is most helpful.

The chakra tradition

Chakra is Sanskrit for wheel. Chakras, also called padmas, or lotuses, form part of the Hindu, Tibetan Buddhist and Chinese spiritual and yogic tradition and in the West were first popularised in the late nineteenth century by the Theosophical movement (see page 10).

As a result of different philosophical emphases, there are considerable variations in the conceptions of the number and function of the chakras. Modern systems usually picture chakras as whirling multi-coloured inverted cones through which the energies pass.

Because they exist on the subtle rather than physical level, chakras cannot be seen or measured physically. Japanese experiments, however, have demonstrated that energy levels in the chakras of people who had worked with chakra energies over a period of years were measurably stronger than those in a control group.

Most traditions locate chakras vertically along the axis of the body, either on or just in front of the backbone; however, they are linked with and take their name from locations on the front of the body, such as the heart, throat and brow. Some researchers and healers, the most notable being the American healer Barbara Ann Brennan, hypothesise that two-sided chakras – similar to double-sided inverted cones – are linked through a central psychic channel, called the *sushumna*. (See page 11 for a method to identify your own chakra points.)

Think of a two-way energy flow from heaven to Earth and Earth to heaven or the body as a pool with two water courses that enter from different places and mingle within it. From above, the universal life force or *prana* is filtered via psychic channels or *nadis* down the chakra system through that lovely soft place which babies have in the centre back of their heads – the fontanelle – before the body has completely closed to the spirit world. As this pure white or golden life force flows in and downwards, each chakra transforms the energy into an appropriate form.

But the energy does not flow through a single channel alone. The same light force is flowing into the individual chakras through the aura all around the body through the chakra connections. This means we are beings of light – it just gets clouded by all the demands of everyday life. If you think of the human body as a broad, flowering tree, the analogy of light flowing in from the cosmos makes more sense.

Just as with the tree whose roots in the ground are essential for its growth and stability, this second source of energy is derived from the Earth and from water that is within or absorbed by the Earth.

Chakra energy itself is said to derive from a latent psychic root energy, called Kundalini-Shakti in Hindu Tantra, and *tumo* in Tibetan Buddhist Tantra. Kundalini is described as a coiled snake sleeping at the base of the spine until activated by meditation, ritual, psychic development, sacred sex or healing work.

A number of practitioners use the minor chakras in the soles of each foot to draw power from the Earth itself to the Root chakra. This triggers the psychic energy and uncoils the Kundalini, herself a manifestation of our repository of Earth power. You may find the foot chakras far easier to work with than the Root chakra itself. This latter is located at the base of the spine or between the genitals and anus – literally our seat of power –

and is a difficult spot because of both anatomical and social restraints in the Western world. In crystal work particularly, the feet, which are ruled by the Root chakra, often form the entry point of empowering and healing energies (see page 117).

The serpent energy travels up the body through the *sushumna*, the central subtle or psychic channel, activating the various chakras. Kundalini is identified with the female energy of Shakti, who is manifest as consort of the Hindu Father God, Shiva in his many forms.

The Shiva energy is the cosmic golden power from above that enters the body through the Crown chakra in the centre of the head.

In addition to the main chakras, some systems recognise more than 120 additional chakra points scattered across the body. Of these, the two in the hands and the two in the feet are perhaps most important for healing work.

The *ida* and *pingala* are the left and right channels that criss-cross the central channel, like the two snakes on the caduceus or staff of Thoth, ancient Egyptian god of learning and medicine. This was later inherited by the Greek Hermes as the symbol for medicine in the Western world (see page 97).

History of the chakras

According to early Eastern chakra tradition, each yogi or adept creates the chakras within his or her body by powerful visualisation and meditative techniques, thereby attaining transcendental awareness. Significantly, chakras are not regarded in this system as independently existing centres within each person, waiting to be activated.

The Hindu Tantric philosophy first developed the concept of chakras. References to life force or *prana* and the *nadis* along which it flows appear in the earliest *Upanishads* or religious books, dating from about 800 BC. The heart was regarded as the centre of 72,000 *nadis*. The later *Upanishads*, dating from the second century BC to the second century AD, refer to chakras per se.

The *Kshurika-Upanishad* mentions the 72,000 *nadis*, identifying the main pathways as well as the central channel, *ida*, the lunar channel and the *pingala*, the solar channel that coil around the *sushumna*. By meditation on the chakras, it was believed that *siddhis* or supernormal powers could be attained by dedicated yogis.

The later and influential Tibetan Buddhist theory of chakras comes from Tantric Buddhism (or Vajrayana) that itself stemmed from the Indian

Tantric tradition. In this system, the power of Kundalini was replaced by the concept of red and white subtle drops of essence in the navel and head chakras.

It was the Western Theosophists who attributed an objective existence to chakras and stated that they could be seen or sensed clairvoyantly. Most influential were W. Leadbeater's books, *The Inner Life* and *The Chakras*. Once these had been published, each of the seven main chakras became regarded as an energy regulator/consciousness transformer, linking the seven subtle spirit or auric bodies. Therefore, the effective functioning of each chakra became associated with the physical and mental as well as the spiritual well-being of the individual.

Finally came the Rainbow theory of chakras, put forward in the early 1970s in Christopher Hill's book *Nuclear Evolution*. Hill stated that each of the chakras corresponds to one of the seven colours of the spectrum. From this point virtually every book on chakra theory has incorporated this concept.

The best of the modern theories retain the connections with the ancient systems, one of which, as outlined below, is based on seven chakras, incorporating different levels of consciousness. Each of the chakras has its own element, symbolic creature, colour, sound, areas and organs of the body, which can be used to strengthen and heal the chakras.

Using this book

Each chapter explores different aspects of the chakras, suggesting ways you can diagnose and heal imbalances physically, emotionally and spiritually. It also suggests the different strengths that can be used to improve your everyday world and gives ways in which you can work with your own unique path of spiritual evolution. Throughout are exercises, rituals, healing ways and empowerments so that you can work not only with your own chakras, but also with those of family and friends. Eventually, if you wish, you can make chakras part of any diagnostic, clairvoyant or therapeutic work you carry out professionally. The first chapter, The Rainbow Body, gives an overview of the seven main chakras and links them with the aura and the different planes of existence. You may find it helpful to begin a chakra journal, noting most crucially your own feelings and insights and also any herbs, incenses, oils or crystals that you use, and any rituals or visualisation work that you carry out.

Exercise to trace your energy patterns

We each have a unique chakra path and it is important to trust your own intuitive awareness more than any book or teacher. This exercise, therefore, relies entirely on your instinctive connection to your energy flows using a crystal pendulum that is perhaps the single most important item you will need for chakra development and healing in yourself and others. Keep a note of your findings and as you learn more you will be amazed by the accuracy of this initial exploration.

If you are already experienced in chakra work, allow your mind to go blank, perhaps by visualising it full of stars. Watch each star go out in turn, until you are left with only velvet darkness.

Let your pendulum trace the energy path as though for the first time. You may be surprised at the insights you receive as a traveller on a path that is familiar in daylight, but suddenly transformed by the mysteries of night.

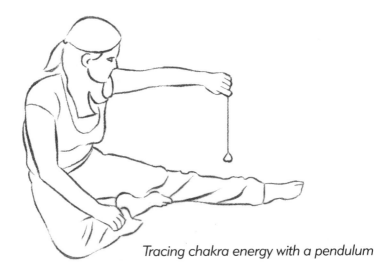

Tracing chakra energy with a pendulum

- Hold the pendulum in your power hand, the one you use for writing, about 2 cm (1 in) away from your body.

- Begin at your left foot and trace an energy path upwards through your body to your head and then down again out of your right foot.

- Let it trace its own path upwards in front of your body, down the right arm and hand, and then up the left hand and arm.

- You may feel a sensation in your fingers like that when you hold your hand over the plug hole of an emptying bath. This is a chakra.

- Other strong energies may occur in the areas of the main internal organs, for example directly over your heart. The sensation has been described as a warm, vibrating drumbeat.

- Allow the pendulum to descend down your spine, spiralling again to the right foot.

- The pendulum may swing gently in a clockwise direction as it follows its spiralling path and anti-clockwise if it reaches a blockage or knot.

- The pendulum may also feel heavy, seem to vibrate out of rhythm or become stuck at one of these points of negative energy.

- If you encounter a knot or blockage, circle the pendulum gently anti-clockwise until you feel the tension loosening.

- If you lose the energy source, perhaps indicated by the pendulum ceasing to swing or the crystal ceasing to buzz, retrace your path to the place where you last felt it. If this area lacks power, energise it with clockwise rotations of the pendulum. Healing and diagnosis go hand in hand in chakra work.

- You may be aware of colours around you at certain points of your body that you may see internally with your clairvoyant or mind's vision.

- Cleanse your pendulum or crystal by plunging it into clear water, preferably in sunlight, shaking off the water and allowing it to dry naturally. This action will both empower and cleanse it.

- Draw an outline of your body in your chakra journal. Mark in the approximate path the pendulum took, the location of chakras, large and small, which can be differentiated by the intensity of the swirling energy, and any blockages and colours you saw.

- This is a good exercise to carry out weekly or when working with the chakras of others for the first time to trace their unique energy flows. As you learn more, you will be able to fine-tune your impressions, but the intuitive information is invariably correct and however much you know or learn, it should always be your base line.

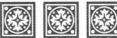

ONE

The Rainbow Body

Each of the chakras is related to one of the colours of the rainbow. These colours, created by the whirling of the chakras, are reflected as bands of colour in the aura, the psychic energy field around each one of us (see pages 14–22).

The brightness and luminosity of the colours reflected in the chakras and the aura, which can be seen clairvoyantly, reveal an individual's state of health and harmony (see page 22 for a quick method of reading the aura and chakras).

By *seeing* the total picture of chakras and aura, you can deduce whether there is a general lack of energy or whether one particular area is blocked, dull and murky, causing another to go into overdrive and perhaps seem particularly harsh or jagged.

At certain times in our lives, all our energies may, temporarily, operate primarily through one chakra. For example, the yellow Solar Plexus energy, stemming from the chakra seated between the navel and the chest, may predominate during a period of intense concentration or when career matters are to the fore. However, if someone lives permanently primarily through this mind and willpower chakra, then the chakra of the Heart or the lower Sacral chakra that deals with love and relationships may become blocked or work only ineffectively. What is more, if red Root energy is not rising to fuel the mind power, then energy stores will become depleted and the person may become exhausted, unable to relax and eventually concentration will disappear.

So chakra work, whether for yourself or others, is a holistic process. Whether you are working in a therapy situation or helping a friend or family member to harmonise their chakra system, talking about the current situation and demands on time and energy can help to set these psychic observations in context and suggest ways in which particular chakras as well as the whole system might be strengthened to make it easier to cope with the everyday world.

In the exercise in the introductory chapter, you sensed the energy flow using a pendulum. On pages 22 and 136 I suggest ways in which you can use clairvoyance and 'clairsentience', which literally mean clear or psychic sight and awareness, to interpret the chakra colours you see.

Because chakras are part of an interconnected system, it is necessary to learn a little about the aura and its different levels in order to have the necessary tools to work with the energy centres themselves.

The seven main chakras

A chapter is devoted to each chakra, but here I will give a brief summary of each, so that you can see the driving force and foci of the rainbow body and its surrounding aura.

In Hindu tradition, the chakras do not have precise anatomical correlations. It was not until the time of the Theosophists that firm links were made between individual chakras and specific endocrine glands and ganglions or plexuses in the sympathetic nervous system.

The Theosophical concept is that workings of the chakras are mirrored in the physical body through the activity of the various glands and nerve plexuses. Because there is disagreement between systems and therefore confusion about precisely which chakra controls which physical area and because of a lack of precise medical knowledge into the workings of glands and nerves, listing precise gland/chakra correlations may be counter-productive. I feel that when we try to tie down psychic concepts and place them into a medical or material framework, we impose artificial limits and that without precise medical knowledge and training, spiritual healing becomes a quasi-science, rather than the free flow of the life force that can find its own path through the body without our intervention once psychic locks are removed. I have, however, listed books on page 155 where you can read about the glands and nerves in relation to chakras, but be sure to use a medical dictionary for precision.

In practice, the chakra energies overlap considerably and in your healing work you can pick up the energies of minor chakras. The key to chakra work is to go with what you find, not what this or any book says you ought to find. If you can become sensitised to your own body energies and those of others, then the template that I and other writers give will be a useful tool. For this reason, I would suggest that you begin with the energy fields of those you love or with whom you have a close friendship, because you are already tuned into their wavelength. It is also easier to touch the person and ask at every point what the effect is, as he or she may be able to guide you to the exact spot at which they can feel the warm fluid-like energy circulating (see Chapter Eleven, Chakras and Relationships).

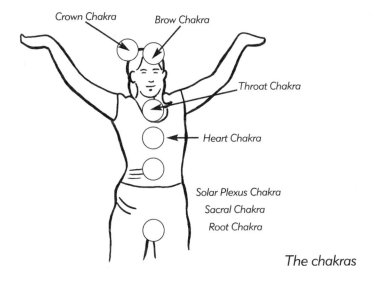

The chakras

The Root chakra

The colour of the Root chakra is red.

You will find the first main chakra at the base of the spine, between the anus and the scrotum or the vaginal cavity and it forms a sphere from the very base of the spine, whose core energy radiates throughout the body. Since this chakra rules the feet and its minor chakras among other body parts, you can work with the feet for contact work such as crystals.

Its function is survival, physical identity, self-preservation and connectedness with our own bodies and with the Earth. Its driving power from the Earth and the Kundalini energy (see page 8) are essential if we are to have the stamina and the basic stability to function effectively and contentedly in the world.

The Root chakra forms the grounding point of the Spirit in the body at birth.

The Sacral chakra

The colour of the Sacral chakra is orange.

You will find the second chakra below the navel in the abdomen around the womb in women and the genitals in men.

Its function is to regulate feelings and desires, including sexuality and to make connections with others. It is concerned with emotional identity, self-esteem and the ability to accept change.

The Solar Plexus chakra

The colour of the Solar Plexus chakra is yellow.

You will find the third chakra above the navel around the stomach area or in some systems further up towards the central cavity of the lungs.

Its function is to galvanise personal power and individuality and to integrate experience. It is concerned with personal identity and setting boundaries, bringing self-confidence and non-aggressive assertiveness.

The Heart chakra

The colour of the Heart chakra is green or pink.

The fourth chakra is located in the centre of the chest and radiates between the upper lung cavity and the heart cavity.

Its function is to facilitate spiritual love between people and a more universal love towards humanity, the earth and all its creatures and the cosmos. It is concerned with inner harmony and specifically with acceptance of the self. It integrates mind and body, self and other, personal and global perspectives and most importantly acts as the transition between the three lower or personal chakras and the higher ones. As this chakra develops, you may become aware of nature spirits and devas, and your own wise ancestors.

The Throat chakra

The colour of the Throat chakra is blue.

The fifth chakra is located in the centre of the throat around the Adam's apple.

Its function is meaningful communication and creativity, and it integrates emotion and thought. It is concerned with self-expression and identity through creativity and is the level upon which symbolism becomes important, especially in dreams and astral travel.

The Third Eye or Brow chakra

The colour of the Brow chakra is indigo.

The sixth chakra is located between and just above the eyes and eyebrows, radiating into the central cavity of the brain.

It aids intuitive insight, psychic functioning and clear-seeing, both in the ability to perceive a wider perspective and clairvoyantly. As integrator of the inner and outer world and other dimensions, it offers contact with angelic or spirit guides and the Higher Self.

The Crown chakra

The colour of the Crown chakra is violet, merging with white or gold as rays from the cosmos pour in.

It is the connection with the cosmic forces and is located at the top of the head, the pivot axis point of the skull, where the different parts of the skull intersect.

Its function is to allow the merging of the individual with cosmic consciousness and connection with the source of divinity through mystical or peak experiences.

This is also the point at which the Spirit enters and leaves the body at birth and death.

The aura and its levels

Each chakra relates to a specific level of the aura. The aura is usually regarded as having seven layers of colour and density, each representing a different layer in the spirit or etheric body that is superimposed upon but also exists within and extends beyond the physical body. Chakras are two-way channels. They energise and colour the aura and the levels of the spirit body as well as the corresponding areas in the physical body. They can in turn be influenced by external factors, for example pollution, people with whom we interact or the burning of a particularly fragrant oil.

At first it may seem confusing that, as well as our physical body, we possess an etheric or spirit body, which can operate independently in out-of-body experiences and which many people think survives death. Obviously, because the two are part of the same system or the physical body is the temple, or less poetically the receptacle, for the spirit body, what affects the one affects the other.

The chakras are psychic not physical entities and exist within the spirit body along the psychic rather than physical spine. Since this is inside the physical body and its energy channels fuel the physical body, we approach, energise, cleanse and heal the chakras directly through the physical body on which they are superimposed. The life force flows in through the chakras and is passed out again to affect the life force within others and the world in this perpetual bi-directional flow.

The colours of the aura are seen in seven bands. The innermost layer, closest to the head and body, is the most dense and is a silvery grey/red in colour.

Of course that silver/red layer is within the body as well but, because the physical body is so dense, matter-wise you cannot see it within the body except clairvoyantly, as a mist. You can, however, see it in the aura, especially around the head where it pops out of the container of the physical body that, maybe owing to a cosmic design fault, just is not big enough for the spirit body that can expand as far as we do spiritually.

This first level or layer of the spirit body corresponds to and is specifically energised by the Root chakra, though of course energies from the other chakras pass down into it.

The other six layers of colour and density are also within the body, but stick out and float even higher above the physical frame. They are superimposed on the red body layer and on the physical body below that, but become less dense and less well formed as we move outwards. However, again you can monitor them in the six outer layers of the aura as it moves from physical body further into the cosmos.

Each of the seven layers is ruled by one of the chakras in ascending order of spirituality. The second, orange body is ruled by the Sacral chakra, which joins the Root layer below and the Solar Plexus layer above. The third, yellow body is ruled by the Solar Plexus chakra, and so on. Once you get to the seventh, violet/white layer that is joined only to the lower, indigo layer fuelled primarily by the Brow chakra, the other side drifts off to merge with cosmic light and energy.

If you were sitting in an aeroplane high up above the world, you would see first the outer violet mist of the highest seventh layer of the body, very misty and ethereal indeed, the stuff the angels and maybe even divinity itself is made of. Then below that is the indigo layer, a little more dense, beneath that the blue, then the green, then the yellow, the orange and the red/silver, each more solid than the one above and finally, beneath them all, terra firma, the physical body.

The chakras too penetrate all seven levels of the spirit, and when you feel their energies with a pendulum or your hands you may be aware that the energy of a single chakra, especially that of a higher chakra, extends beyond the physical body into what makes up the aura. The centre of the Crown chakra, for example, can be felt about three finger-breadths above the physical head (see page 105).

As you evolve spiritually, the energy from the higher or more spiritual chakras becomes available in your daily life and hence the colours with higher vibrations such as blue or indigo will be manifest in your aura. When a particular auric colour appears temporarily to dominate the halo, you know that the corresponding chakra which creates that colour is providing the main energy input, even if generally your chakra and auric rainbow is well balanced.

Initially, it may be easier to read the aura than the chakras, though in time you will be able to see these energy centres psychically as though they were part of your actual physical body, using your psychic ultra sound (see pages 22 and 136).

If, for example, your Heart chakra is particularly evolved and active during a certain period, if you are doing a lot of charitable work or are in a deep and spiritual love relationship, not only will your aura reflect emerald green, the chakra itself will shine particularly brightly in your body around the heart region where it is sited. Ideally you will generally have a perfect rainbow around your head and body as your auric sphere and correspondingly glowing rainbow chakras all work in harmony.

In practice, much therapeutic work takes place on the first three personal levels of the Spirit body/auric levels that correspond with the three lower personal chakras. In many people beyond the third layer of the aura may seem hazy and the upper chakras may move quite slowly. Many people live like that quite happily for all of their lives or until a major crisis causes a life re-assessment. Age too can bring higher chakra functioning through experience. It is important therefore only to offer healing and higher chakra work if a person wants it, even if their life seems unsatisfactory to you.

The three higher layers of the body replicate the three lower bodies but at a higher level of vibration. Some regard these as forming the soul and as the seat of our higher self. When we utilise this level of our being, we can more easily commune with angels and beings of higher spiritual orders, at first in dreams as we expand our consciousness and then more directly.

I shall now describe the seven levels of the aura in turn, but if these seem confusing or are not helpful to you, remember that they are just another way of looking at body energies and you can work with your chakras without referring to them. You will see that the descriptions closely mirror the corresponding chakra functions.

The etheric layer

This first level is fuelled by the Root chakra, and so, when functioning fully, will be seen as red. The overlap of this body extends from 0.5 cm (¼ in) to 5 cm (2 in) beyond the physical body on which it is superimposed, following the outline of the physical form. Its name is confusing since it is the same as that of the whole etheric or spirit body, but it is different and refers here to just one layer.

As the most dense layer of the spirit body with the lowest vibrations and located closest to the physical body, it reflects especially the physical condition of the body.

It is the blueprint for the physical body and so any potential problems will be manifest as darkness, jagged lines, holes or patches of harsh or murky colours relating to one of the other malfunctioning chakras. Because this occurs before physical or mental symptoms appear in the physical body or mind, then it can act as an early warning signal to change lifestyle or reduce stresses as well as reflecting actual physical problems.

The emotional layer

The Sacral chakra controls this second layer which may appear as orange. This layer deals with our emotional reactions (as opposed to the higher interactions of the fourth level) and our desires for love, sex, success, even for food or alcohol as an emotional prop. The emotional layer is usually seen as a swirling mass of energy about the body. It approximates to the outline but is not as clearly defined as the etheric layer. In fact, as we move through the levels, they follow less closely the structure of a physical person.

This is the level most subject to change with emotion. It can also temporarily obscure the other layers.

The mental layer

The Solar Plexus chakra governs the third level of thought and ideas, where thoughts become reality and at which magic takes place. This level is also affected by everyday interactions, though it represents a more measured response than the pure emotions.

This level is usually most visible around the head and shoulders as a yellowish light.

The astral layer

The Heart chakra rules the fourth auric layer that divides the three lower and personally orientated bodies and those that link to higher dimensions.

This is the layer of spiritual love and permanent relationships, driven by consciously directed feelings and not the more random emotions and desires of the second body. It is perceived as green or pink. People who are especially altruistic towards others may also have a pink tinge to the other layers. Once you are operating on this level of vibration, you resonate with the planes of existence inhabited by people who have lived in the past and so you may experience some mediumistic powers and an awareness of past lives and worlds. Healing energies are derived from here, especially those that use natural sources such as herbs or crystals.

The etheric template

The Throat chakra controls this fifth level, which is blue and a copy of the physical body on a spiritual vibration. Some see this level of functioning as triggering awareness of the essential self that enables the spirit body to detach itself in astral or out-of-body travel and which becomes stronger and more active as we move through our lives.

It is at this stage of evolution in chakra work that divination, dreams of other dimensions and clairaudience are manifest as part of our lives. For this is a level at which the collective unconscious or cosmic memory bank can be accessed and the boundaries of time lose their meaning.

You may need to work with your chakras for several months before being able to access this level easily and regularly. But the reward for this effort is to see the blue healing light in your permanent aura that typifies healers who draw on higher energies.

The celestial body

The Third Eye or Brow chakra fuels this sixth layer that forms the body of emotional level on the spiritual plane. Its colour is indigo.

Emotions are now homed into global concerns and tuned also to the world of light beings, angels and Archangels.

After a year or so of chakra work, you may start to function regularly at this level. You may find your channelling abilities, perhaps through automatic writing or psychic artistry, evolve, as do prophetic abilities.

The ketheric template

The Crown chakra controls this seventh layer and it may take several years before you are sufficiently spiritually evolved to work fully with these energies. At this level you can merge with the cosmic energies and you may experience direct momentary awareness of the source of divinity. It is the stage at which if we do grow in wisdom as our years on earth increase, we can hope to step off the karmic wheel and understand the wider purpose of the universe. For many people this stage is realised at the point of death: the dying person reports brilliant light and subsequently relatives may see the spirit leaving the body as pure white light.

The colour of this level is violet merging to white or gold.

Reading the aura and chakras

You may initially wish to begin to read the coloured halo around the body, but you may find that you can also see or sense clairvoyantly chakra colours within the body, as well as around specific organs.

The method below is just a technique to make a start with and, as you work more with chakra energies, your innate clairvoyance will enable you to see colours around everyone and everything.

Since this ability resides not in the physical but the psychic eye, you have to learn to de-activate the conscious, analytical part of the mind and allow your psychic vision that is ruled by the Third Eye chakra to emerge; it will do this quite spontaneously. The hardest part is not *seeing* but in trusting what you see with your inner eye or sense.

I have used and taught this method many times for aura reading. After a time, once you gain confidence in your ability, you can usually *see* circles of colour within the body. This sensation is, as I said earlier in the chapter, rather like looking down through the holes in clouds from a plane and seeing houses or trees below.

However, if you prefer to read the colours of the auric bands alone, you can do so and the results will be one and the same.

The easiest way I find is to look either at yourself in a mirror or a subject framed against light (you may prefer the subject with a darker background, so experiment). Some people say that what you are aware of is an after-image, but in fact you are not using a physical sensation at all except as an entry point. Whatever is happening physiologically is like the engine in a car that is necessary for a car to work, but has little to do with the prowess of the driver or the nature of the scenery through which you are passing.

- Draw the outline of a body – don't worry about layers.

- Have a set of coloured pencils ready with at least three hues for each colour. A box of thirty plus colours is ideal. Watercolours or marker pens may be used, but paints in general do not work as well.

- Look at the area around the head, close your eyes for a few seconds, open them, blink and then you will get a vivid impression of the aura, either externally or in your mind's vision. Both are as good. The red colour will be closest to the head and the outermost violet/white layer may extend up to an arm's span from the innermost layer.

- You may also quite spontaneously become aware of the individual chakra circles of colour within the body. The psyche is like a flashbulb camera and holds intact the instantaneous image.

- Record your impressions quickly, colouring in the aura, chakras and any blobs of colour. Add diagrams or notes as you wish. For example, you may write, 'blue missing, red very harsh through the seven chakras'.

- Write or draw in the way that you do in an examination as time runs out. Do not stop to analyse or rationalise what you are recording, as you will lose the flow. You already trust the evidence of your physical sight, and in time you will come to trust the inner sight that cannot be fooled by tricks of light or memory processes that shape perceptions.

- If you lose concentration, look at the aura again quickly, but allow your hand to pick the correct colours automatically.

- You may have recorded dark lines or streaks, jagged areas or even holes in the aura or a dark haze around a chakra that would indicate a blockage.

- As a general rule a very pale shade or a missing colour needs extra energy related to that chakra to be added. Harshness or jaggedness requires excess negativity to be removed.

- Dull, turgid colours indicate a blockage.

See pages 118–126 for methods of cleansing and healing the chakras and auric field.

Strengthening the auric bodies and chakras

Use this method to increase your awareness of the different energy centres and to strengthen and energise your individual chakras.

- Sit in front of a wide-angled mirror – a free-standing, full-length looking glass is ideal.

- Take seven candles, one in each of the rainbow colours. Arrange these in a diagonal line, starting with the red candle behind and slightly to the side of you. You should be able to see all seven candles in the mirror.

- Light the red candle first, then the orange candle, then, in order, yellow, green, blue, indigo and violet.

- When you can see the candles in a pathway, switch off all other lights and focus first on the red candle.

- Visualise its rays as a swirling hoop of colour close to your body, encircling you, combining the light with your own red auric energies that flow in and out of your red Root chakra, joining the red ellipse on either side of your body. The ellipse will undulate in and out, approximately following the lines of your body.

- For each colour you visualise you may experience different emotions and sensations, and for the outer colours, blue through to violet, you may experience images of higher beings, words or music from the higher planes.

- Continue to focus on each of the colours in turn, moving outwards so that you add to the colour bands whirling around you.

- You may become aware of white light above your head pouring upwards as well as downwards, as the seven rays synthesise as a white halo.

- Sit for a while in the candlelight to strengthen your own aura, leaving you energised but calm.

- Look in the mirror once more and you may be rewarded by luminosity all around you.

- Let the candles burn down in a safe place.

Whenever you experience difficulty in studying your own auric levels or those of someone else, recall the candles to your mind.

Repeat this ritual about once a month to keep your chakras healthy and to strengthen your auric vision. As you become more experienced, change the emphasis from the auric bands to the seven chakras within you. You will almost instantly become aware of the rainbow body within.

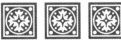

TWO

Working with the Individual Chakras

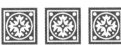

The following seven chapters examine each of the chakras in detail and suggest ways you can help them to function more effectively and so benefit from their specific energies in your life. Work through the sections in order and try those activities that seem relevant before moving on to the next level.

There may be certain chakras that you wish to explore more fully because they relate to areas of your life that are significant at a particular time.

You can return to any of the chakra exercises at times when you need their energies or if you sense the energy is not flowing freely. Moving upwards through the chakras is not a once-and-for-all progression, but a circuit in which the energy flow moves constantly upwards and downwards in harmony.

You may find it helpful to read through the next seven chapters quickly and, if you wish, the rest of the book before returning to the detailed work on the separate chakras.

If you are new to the subject, you may need a week or so to familiarise yourself with chakra energies. Start by concentrating on the Root chakra but, as you progress, you may want to work on developing two chakras at the same time, perhaps beginning study of a new one while continuing rituals for the previous one. Sometimes as you develop a new chakra, the work you carried out on a lower chakra suddenly takes on a different perspective. Alternatively, you may want to apply a higher-level technique to overcome blocks you experienced in earlier chakra work. If you are already experienced, you may find alternative approaches that can give fresh impetus to your ongoing spiritual development.

Your energy system is unique. There are no rights and wrongs, no rules, no timetables or set steps. At the end of this section, however, I have listed two basic techniques, meditation and sacred sound that can be used to empower and harmonise all the chakras individually and together. If these do not work for you, there are many other equally valid ways of tuning into your chakra energies.

Remember how you learned to drive a car or ride a bike. At first there seemed so much to remember but, in time, the process becomes automatic. In the same way, you will find that you can attune your chakras while squashed in a crowded commuter train or standing in the supermarket queue.

Creating a special place for chakra work

You can work with your chakras absolutely anywhere. As with any natural energies, however, the open air offers instant contact with the same powers that flow through all natural energy fields.

However, if you do create a special place in which to spend your chakra time and where you can gather all the materials you will need, the place, the materials and above all you, will accumulate the positive energies over days, weeks and months. Here you will be able to move easily from the everyday world into your personal spiritual realm. Here too you can come when you feel tired or stressed and sit quietly in natural light or with a candle, allowing the powers of the place to take away pain and tension, so that your energies flow more freely.

This need not be elaborate. A table in the corner of a quiet room, a conservatory, summer house or attic will do. In better weather, use a secluded spot in a garden or on a balcony where you can improvise with a large tree stump or slab of stone supported by rocks – even a picnic table and benches. As well as my more permanent place in the room in which I now write, I have a small box of chakra materials which I place on the table outside my caravan. I can then work under the pine trees, away from the demands of family, neighbours and people who desperately want to sell me double-glazing.

You can keep a box or chest with candles and crystals of the seven different colours and special treasures associated with each chakra so that when you need the energies of a specific chakra, you can fill the table with its related crystals, incenses etc.

At other times you may take out the artefacts associated with two or three chakras – or even all seven – to harmonise and empower the whole system. You can buy statues or pictures of the chakra deities or angels or download images from the Internet or display flowers or branches from the different chakra trees (a list of correspondences is given in the individual chakra chapters).

Your chakra journal

Because chakras are so personal and so relevant to every aspect of life, you may find it helpful to keep a personal journal of your psychic exploration of the energy field. Each chakra will invoke different emotions and ideas, and your meditation and visualisation work will create images and visions the significance of which will unfold over the days after the experience (see page 29). You may find that, as the weeks progress, you are writing poetry or stories of the fabulous creatures inspired by the different chakra animals or that you begin to paint or draw the rainbow visions you see or sense, even if previously you felt you had little ability or inclination.

If you buy a loose-leaf folder, you can add charts of chakra readings you carry out for yourself and others, and details of any healing or empowering work with perhaps additional readings taken after individual healing sessions to monitor progress.

You can also record auras you see around yourself and others that will also over time reflect any chakra healing or strengthening rituals you carry out.

As you work with the higher chakras, you can record any especially significant dreams, telepathic links, astral or past-life travel and channelling received from devas or angelic beings.

You can add images or your own artistic impressions of the chakra deities and angels, plus rituals that you have created as a result of reading and adapting mine.

Like any diary, your chakra journal will reflect your spiritual and creative evolution and as you re-read the earlier pages, you will be surprised how far you have travelled.

Chakra correspondences

Chakra energies are triggered by and manifest in different forms throughout the natural world, for example in specific crystals or herbs associated with each chakra centre.

These natural materials can be used to open specific chakra points, clear blockages and direct the inherent chakra powers into everyday life or for spiritual development. Though some people work purely with inner processes such as meditation and visualisation, for many of us, tangible objects on which to focus make it easier to link in with the specific energies of each chakra and enhance our inner explorations.

Some materials are especially powerful. Crystals, because of their own vibrant energy field (see pages 118–122), can be applied directly to chakra points, used as a focus for absent healing, empowered and carried or worn as talismans to release the strengths inherent in their ruling chakra. They can also be soaked in pure spring water which is then drunk, splashed on pulse points or added to bath water so that the body can absorb the chakra energies.

Rainbow-coloured light is inhaled from different coloured candles according to the chakra power that is desired. This energy can also be absorbed from living sources that are especially rich in *prana* or the life force, such as flowers or fruit.

The planetary deities, gods and goddesses and archangels associated with the various energy centres can be invoked in chakra rituals or in mantras to open individual chakras.

Herbs, flowers and leafy twigs from associated trees can be placed in your special chakra place while you are working with a specific chakra, burned as incense or oils (see pages 122–125), made into smudge sticks or added to baths.

The sacred geometric symbol and creatures representing the strengths of each chakra can be used as amulets or in meditation.

The suggested activities for awakening each chakra can be easily incorporated into your daily life if necessary, but can also be developed during your private times away from the demands of the world. Because the chakra system is interconnected, when you work with one chakra, the benefits spread to the others. Equally, when you open a chakra, healing and balancing are part of the process, as is strengthening, so the terms are usually interchangeable.

Meditation

Meditation means, quite simply, to focus on one thought, idea, sound or image while excluding all other thoughts and actions. Its purpose is to create the inner stillness and silence, like the space between two waves or, in the Zen Buddhist analogy, like one hand clapping.

If all you have is five or ten minutes a day meditating in your special chakra place, using one of the associated foci, you will find that any blockages are released and that the energy flows not only through the selected chakra, but through the whole system.

Some people find the idea of meditating daunting. If you have ever closed your eyes by a fountain and listened to the water, lain in sunlit grass with the breeze gently moving the stalks, looked, half-asleep, from a plane window on mile after mile of cotton wool clouds, or listened to bees humming on a drowsy summer day and seemed to understand what they were saying, you have already meditated. The most successful instant method I have encountered is to picture a sky full of stars and watch them one by one going out until you are enclosed in a velvety blackness (see page 107).

A *formal method of chakra meditation*

- In your special place, indoors or out, light one of your chakra fragrances as incense (see page 123). There are special garden incense sticks available.

- If you are lying down, be sure your back and neck are properly supported, with your arms loosely by your side and hands lightly touching the bed or couch.

- If you are sitting, place both feet flat on the floor. You may, if you wish, support your back with a pillow and have armrests on the chair for your elbows. Rest your arms comfortably in your lap, with palms facing upwards.

- Some people prefer to sit cross-legged on the floor with their hands supporting their knees. If you practise yoga, use the lotus position, although this means your feet will not touch the ground.

- Place your chakra focus, for example a sacred shape, a god/dess statue or image, a large chakra crystal or flower, so that you can see it without moving your neck or head. You can create a set of large chakra geometric symbols on stiff card for meditation.

- Concentrate on your breathing, inhaling light and exhaling darkness so that you and the symbol are enclosed in light.

- Take slow deep breaths through your nose, hold them for a count of three and slowly exhale through your nose again. (Some people use external rhythmic sound, for example a metronome or a recording of waves rising and falling, to set the pace of their breathing.) Repeat this until your breathing is slow and steady.

- Become your breathing and do not attempt to move beyond it. Keep focused on the external stimulus either by looking at it or by closing your eyes and visualising the stimulus in your mind's eye.

- Let the internal or external focus expand and fill your mind, so that all other sights, sounds and sensations recede.

- Hold the image for about five minutes, letting the colour and energies of the object merge with your energies and the colour of the related chakra within you, so that you are the focus and it is you. You may be aware of increased colour or warm liquid flowing through you and may see images or hear words.

- Accept but do not try to develop or rationalise them for they are part of the experience, related to the chakra with which you are working.

- Gradually move away from the focus, letting the image or thought fade, connecting with your breathing and letting the light also fade. As you do this, external sounds will return and your normal range of vision will expand.

- If you closed your eyes, open them slowly, blinking and stretching slowly like a cat uncurling after sleep.

Mantras

Throughout the ages, in almost every religion, formal as well as natural, chanting, singing and rhythm have offered a pathway to raise consciousness and enter mystical trance states.

Since only a small proportion of the vibrations of the universe can be heard by the human ear, the purpose of chant and song is to attune the spirit of the chanter or musician to the more subtle sounds on higher levels. In doing so, it is said, the soul will move closer to harmony and finally unity with the cosmic rhythms – and the *sound of silence*.

Chanting thus offers a perfect way to align and harmonise the chakras. In the following chapters I have listed a sacred sound associated with each chakra. However, you can create your own chants, based around the basic affirmation of the power of the individual chakra.

In the mantras that I have given the 'a' is always soft, like the 'u' in 'sun'; the 'm' is long, as in 'mother'.

The mantra should follow the natural outflow of breath. When the sounds are made silently, in the mind, the mantra should be repeated on the in and the out breath. Sometimes a mantra is said out loud to begin with, then silently with the silence being longer. Some people whisper mantras so that they can be heard by them alone. You may find it easier to exhale through your mouth when chanting aloud.

In meditation, once you have established your breathing pattern, you can close your eyes and recite a simple chant over and over, either aloud or in your mind. It does not matter how trite the mantra seems, the idea is to establish the mesmeric rhythm that gradually fades into silence and is heard in your head. In the same way that you became the focus in your meditation, you can merge with the sound.

Mantras can also be written down to make patterns (see page 88).

Chakra sound and colour

Each chakra has its own musical note on the scale. A simple way of opening your chakras and clearing blockages is to sing the scale slowly upwards while visualising the rainbow light rising from red through to violet.

- You can also visualise the chakra circles expanding and turning clockwise as you activate them with the sound.

- Go down the scale slowly to close the chakras temporarily if you need to protect yourself from hostility or confrontation or if your mind is whirling and you need to sleep. Singing in your head is a good instant and unobtrusive form of psychic protection.

- For energising the system, go up and down the scale several times, ending at the top of the scale, singing either the colour names as shown overleaf, the chakra names, or doh, ray, me etc.

- If the energies within you feel sluggish or you need a sudden surge of energy or courage, you can increase the speed as you sing. You can also sing in a round with a lover, friend or family member, each beginning a note behind the other.

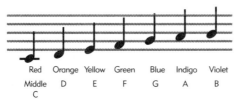

Red	Orange	Yellow	Green	Blue	Indigo	Violet
Middle C	D	E	F	G	A	B

Music and chant work is especially potent in work with the Throat chakra, the elemental ruler of which is sound (see pages 77–88).

THREE

The Root Chakra
or Muladhara

The Root chakra is the foundation of the entire chakra system as well as the home of the individual human spirit as it moves into the world and takes on a physical body. On the Isle of Wight where I live we suffer from landslips and subsidence and, while stripping the walls to decorate my house, I found some rather disturbing cracks, suggesting that my home may soon need underpinning to secure the foundations. Just as a building needs secure foundations and a tree needs strong roots to survive the tests of time and weather so, if we are to feel secure and comfortable within ourselves, we need a well-functioning core or Root chakra. It is no use just papering over the cracks.

Security is far more than putting money into a building society account or accumulating material goods. It is feeling comfortable within yourself, as you are, where you are. It encompasses the ability to withstand the pressures of life without being ruled by the flight-or-fight mechanism, and not to constantly veer between elation and despair and back again. It is the ability to accept and succeed within the limitations of the real world, not to fritter our time and resources on unattainable dreams or be so afraid of failing that we never paddle out beyond the shallows of life. Self-esteem and power will be explored in the next two chapters, but they definitely have their roots here. The Root chakra, then, is not dull, but the vessel in which we can sail to far-off places in actuality and spiritually, secure that home is still waiting when we grow tired of voyaging.

Location of the Root chakra

This is the chakra of the Earth and it draws its beautiful deep red light upwards from the Earth, through the feet, and through our perineum when we sit on the ground. Both of these are points at which the Root chakra can be accessed and healed. The minor chakras in the soles of the feet are also ruled by and connected directly to the Root.

The Root chakra rules the legs, feet and skeleton including the teeth and the large intestine.

Imbalances can be reflected as pain and tension in any of these, as constipation or irritable bowel symptoms, a general lack of energy and an inability to relax even when exhausted. On a psychological level, unreasonable anger or paralysing fear from trivial causes can be a symptom of a blockage. As well as the work in this section, see Chapter Ten on healing.

Kundalini, the goddess within

Coiled at the base of the spine around the perineum in every man, woman and child lies the individual manifestation of the goddess Kundalini. Both a Hindu and universal goddess, Kundalini is the serpent power. This is our inner source of Earth and transformative power that enables us to rise upwards spiritually and mentally, like a magnificent swaying cobra, a beautiful tall building or a magnificent tree to touch the sky, knowing that we are firmly held by Mother Earth and so cannot fall.

Kundalini is associated with the female polarity of the Shakti or Mother Goddess energy that activates Shiva, the Father Sky, the creative force that enters the body through the Crown chakra in the centre of the head (see pages 103–116). In Tantra, a Hindu system of spirituality, the core of which is sacred sex, sexual energy is used to ignite the Kundalini, and in Chapter Twelve I explore sexual power and bliss through activating the chakra system. As you work with your chakras, however, this energy will unfold spontaneously and fill you with the surging energy of the Earth that lies just beneath the crust.

This then is a very special chakra, the beginning of the journey and, for our bodies, also the end as we return to the womb of the Mother while our spirit returns to the cosmos.

This is the Mother chakra, first awakened when our own mother holds us and feeds us as an infant. As we work at strengthening this chakra we shall meet the wise Earth goddesses and Saturn or Old Father Time to keep us on track. Working with the Earth energies will help us to connect with that source of power we sometimes lose sight of in high-rise buildings and urban streets. For if we can symbolically embed ourselves in the Earth and our spirits firmly in our bodies, we can learn the lessons we were sent into this world to discover and use our Root powers to connect or reconnect with our higher spiritual nature. For westernised chakra work is firmly embedded in the principle not of escaping from this life into a state of undifferentiated cosmic bliss, but of enjoying every possible moment of sunshine and bringing the spiritual into the everyday world.

Root chakra correspondences

As I said in the previous chapter, you can use the chakra correspondences in ways limited only by your imagination. As you work through this chapter, you may wish to create a Root chakra centre in your special place.

Colour

Red is associated with the Root chakra.

You can begin by lighting a red candle and sitting quietly in your special place, watching the flame through half-closed eyes and visualising the red, whirling Root chakra and the rich red and golden earth.

Visualise yourself breathing in red light from the candle or from red flowers that grow in your region, and gently exhale darkness. Eat or drink raw or unprocessed red foods, such as redcurrants, red apples or raspberry juice.

Element

The element related to the Root chakra is Earth.

Walk across grass or sand barefoot, dig your toes into the soil and sand. Make sandcastles and dance on the beach or in your garden when no one is around. Allow your feet to follow the spiralling rhythm pulsating within the soil and sand, especially at ancient sites.

Work with clay, allowing it to form and reform into pots, figures, Earth and serpent goddess figures or animals, especially those associated with this chakra as listed below. You can display them in your special place.

In Africa, in an unbroken tradition over thousands of years, pots have great magical significance as representations and containers of the life-giving powers of the potter and, through her, the Great Mother. Pregnant women, however, are not allowed to make pots because they already have demands on their fertility and it is feared that too much of their creative energy will flow into the pots instead of the unborn child. Only men or post-menopausal women are permitted to decorate pots with animals or human figures, as such an activity could compromise a fertile woman's creative power.

Work also with wood, another Root chakra material, smoothing fallen twigs and branches and creating shapes, god or goddess forms or animals with them. In some African traditions, woodcarving carries the same taboos about female creativity. But in the modern westernised world, women, as well as men, find wood and clay work, simple or complex, connects them to the Root energy – a connection that we have lost because of the nature of urban life. Anyone can create beautiful things with as simple a tool as a penknife, and your abstract creation will hold endless possibilities for future interpretation.

Symbols

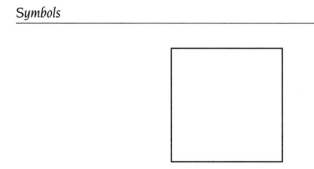

The red square and spiral are the symbols of the Root chakra.

The square symbolises energy that is contained within and can be channelled through time and space. You can use this symbol in meditation or paint a square on a red crystal to serve as an amulet.

The spiral is another sacred shape associated with this chakra. It often appears as a coiled snake and is one of the earliest and most widespread goddess motifs, being found in the art of the American Indians, Australian Aborigines, Asian and European cultures. A spiral shell is a good focus, as are twisted twigs and branches. You can also decorate your pots with spirals, as people have done for thousands of years.

Mantra sound

Lam (pronounced Lu-u-um) is the mantra sound related to the Root chakra.

You can use this sound for meditation, tap it out on a drum or chant it as you dance. Alternatively create your own power mantra for this chakra.

Planet ♄

The planet of the Root chakra is Saturn.

As the shadow side of the Sky God Jupiter who rules the Brow chakra, Saturn is the reality factor, the constraints of fate, time and space. But he can also turn challenge into opportunity through effort and perseverance. Saturnus is the Roman form of Cronus, Greek God of Time, and was deposed by his son Jupiter, after he had refused to allow natural change and progression. But even this led to joy, because Saturnus was sent to Italy where he taught the farmers agriculture and engineering, establishing a Golden Age of peace and plenty.

Saturn rules Capricorn (22 December–20 January) and is co-ruler of Aquarius (21 January–18 February).

These Sun periods are most potent for Root chakra work and those born under these signs will relate to this chakra most easily.

Saturday, Saturn's day, is especially good for all Root chakra work.

Find out all you can about Saturn by reading and loading images from the Internet.

Like all the pagan gods, Saturn had a dark as well as a creative side – part of the reality principle is that we all have a shadow side. Confronting and channelling negativity is an important part of working with our roots.

A very dark blue or brown candle is good for working with Saturn energies.

Archangel

Cassiel is the angel of the Root chakra.

Though Cassiel, the conservator, is called the angel of solitude and temperance, he was traditionally invoked for investment and speculation. In one sense, this is not incompatible, for true speculation is based not on an uncoordinated random process, but on deliberation and an almost intuitive scanning of any situation. He brings moderation in actions and dealings, and development of inner stillness and contemplation.

Though channelling is associated with the highest two chakras (Brow and Crown), you can work with angel energies at this level. This is because the entire chakra system is interlinked and so angelic powers will filter down to the lower chakras, though, for example, the Root chakra angel may be primarily manifest as a guardian who offers advice on practical issues and offers the protection of a loving parent. Find information on and images of Cassiel on the Internet or in books (see page 155).

Invoke Cassiel in a red or deep blue or brown candle and allow images and wise words to form in your mind. For this and your Saturn work, light an incense associated with this chakra and hold one or more of your chakra crystals to make contact with these energies. (See page 39 for the correct incense and crystals to use.) Record your insights and any messages in your chakra journal.

Deities

All Earth and serpent goddesses are associated with the Root chakra.

In Neolithic times the goddess was pictured in various cultures and under different names with snakes entwining or close to her body. This image continued through the Classical world, but was progressively demonised as the Father gods became supreme.

In Hindu myth, between incarnations, Brahma, the creator god, and other gods slept on the coils of the world serpent goddess *shesha* or Ananta, goddess of infinite time. She is identified with the goddess Kundalini.

Or you might prefer an Earth goddess. My favourite is the Australian Aboriginal creator woman Warramurrungundjui who emerged from the sea and gave birth to the first people. She is an amazingly practical creatrix, for she carried a digging stick and a bag of food plants, medicinal plants and flowers. Having planted these, she went on to dig the necessary water holes and then, leaving her children to enjoy the fruits of her work, she turned herself into a rock.

Throughout the myths of many Native North American nations runs the symbol of Grandmother Spider Woman, the female creative principle who wove the web of the world, taught wisdom and various crafts to her people and even protected them from bad dreams with her dreamcatchers.

In Hopi myth, Spider Woman and Tawa, the Sun deity, created the Earth between them. With magical songs from the thoughts and images in

Tawa's mind, Spider Woman fashioned from clay wonderful animals, birds and finally man and woman. Men and women were given life as Spider Woman cradled them in her arms and Tawa blew his warm breath over them.

There are countless serpent and Earth goddesses: enter the words on an Internet search engine and the legends come alive.

You may like to collect Mother Goddess statues or make your own. Most towns have museums displaying such artefacts. One rich source is the British Museum in London, though I much prefer the Museum of Cluny on the Left Bank in Paris with its amazing array of Black Madonnas, the Christianised Earth Mother, who may be seen laughing with and breastfeeding her child.

Creatures

The bull, serpent, dragon and snake are related to the Root chakra.

The bull is the male Root chakra sign. It is an icon that appears in early Neolithic art of the Earth Mother giving birth to a bull or horned god figure as her son and consort. Bull dances and bull sacrifices, the origin of the bull fight, were performed in honour of the Mother Goddess in Crete and in pre-Christian times in other Mediterranean lands such as Spain, where the vestiges have survived.

Serpents or dragons are also symbols of the Root chakra Earth goddesses. Visit animal parks or farms where you can see these creatures. There are many large lizards that bear dragon characteristics.

The dragon myth can be found from the Middle East to Central America. Originally the dragon was a representation of the Earth Mother. Dragon-slaying myths have evolved to represent the struggle to defeat Mother Goddess worship, and Christianity has many examples of dragon-slaying saints – female as well as male. In the oriental world, however, dragons were said to hold the secrets of the Earth and to guard rich treasure.

The ability of the snake to shed its skin gave rise to legends that it was immortal and indeed the icon of the snake Ouroboros swallowing its own tail became, in alchemical symbolism, a representation of eternity. You may choose to make a snake out of a small branch. Choose one that has bark attached and, as you whittle away the bark with a knife or special tool obtained from a craft shop, name and shed the redundant angers or fears in a chant such as:

Banish the anger, drive away pain, fall away fear, make me free again.

All these creatures can be used in meditation.

Crystals

Bloodstone, garnet, red jasper, lodestone, obsidian, smoky quartz, ruby, and black tourmaline are the crystals corresponding to the Root chakra.

All of these can be circled over your Root chakra area or placed on your feet to connect you with the power of the Earth (see page 119 for a chakra crystal ritual). You can also paint chakra symbols on the crystals or carry them unadorned in a tiny red purse or drawstring bag to give you physical energy, courage, strength and security at difficult times in your life.

Use a large piece of smoky quartz as a focus for meditation and to transmit images as you sit by candlelight in your special place.

Incenses and oils

Cypress, ivy, mimosa, patchouli, tea tree and vetivert are all associated with the Root chakra.

Burn these during Root chakra work and at any time in your home to settle the atmosphere. This will also purify the air after quarrels and attract abundance into your home and faithful relationships into your life.

Herbs

Aconite, basil, bistort, comfrey, horsetail and Solomon's seal are associated with the Root chakra.

Use dried herbs, and empower them by mixing them in a ceramic or wooden bowl with a ceramic or wooden spoon, while stating the specific purpose as a mantra, for example:

Banish fear, anxiety clear, courage appear.

Chant the words over and over again faster and faster, visualising red light pouring upwards from the Earth.

Place the empowered herbs with a chakra crystal in a red purse. Carry this with you or keep it under your pillow until the particular aspect of the Root is strengthened or the crisis past. You can also use the oils and incenses listed above in their herb form (see page 156 for herb books listing specific properties).

Trees

The trees associated with the Root chakra are the aspen, blackthorn, cypress, poplar, redwood and yew.

All trees have especially strong associations with the Root chakra and you can derive energy by sitting beneath them, hugging them or dancing around them, either alone or with friends. The trees just listed are especially effective. The following ritual is one I find helpful for harmony and healing of fear or anger.

- Sit at the foot of your chosen tree facing the direction of the sun with your back against the trunk.

- Let the energies of the tree enter you via the base of your spine at the Root chakra.

- Visualise the rich golden red light and warmth rising through the roots of the tree and following the energy channels of your body, circulating through every nadir and channel and flowing down again, like a huge wave, so that you are the tree.

- When the energies have flowed back, draw up more and this time see them warming and awakening the coiled snake, the Kundalini, who slowly uncoils and gently sends the energies spiralling upwards, so that you feel alive and connected with, but not overwhelmed by, the energy.

- If this feels too powerful, visualise some of the power flowing down into the roots again.

- Walk or run, barefoot if possible, and extend your arms so that you are also drawing in the power of the sunshine – or even rain.

- Whenever you feel tired or worried, return to your special tree. If this is not always possible, make a tiny wooden amulet from a twig from the tree so that by touching it you can recall the power.

- If none of the Root trees listed grows in your region, then find a tree that has deep roots and symbolises strength to you.

Affirmation

'I am' is the affirmation corresponding to the Root chakra.

You can use this as a basis for chants that you can recite or sing, for example:

I am, I am wo/man,

Therefore I can.

Working with the Root chakra

The easiest way to earth or ground yourself is to stand barefoot on grass or earth.

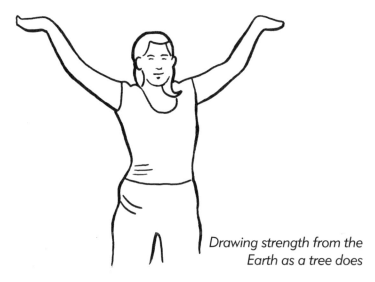

Drawing strength from the Earth as a tree does

- Raise your hands above your head while breathing in; then, fingers extended, slowly lower them down towards the Earth while breathing out. At the end of the movement your arms should be by your sides with the fingers pointing to the Earth.

- Press your feet hard down on the ground. Visualise yourself exhaling darkness slowly and feel the darkness flowing into the soil where it will be recycled into positivity.

- If you are feeling afraid or angry, stamp your feet, saying:

It is gone, it is done, peace come.

- Alternatively, sit on the ground and raise your arms, then press down with your hands, feet and perineum.

- When you feel free, you can then reverse the process, drawing red light through the roots of the Earth into your perineum. Again extend your arms and this time inhale the rich red and golden brown light of the Earth.

- For those times when you cannot go outdoors, keep a living plant nearby. Bury two dark-coloured Root crystals in the soil. Very gently touch the plant and close your eyes, running your fingers through the soil, allowing what the mediaeval mystic Hildegard von Bingen called the greening process, to reconnect you with the Earth.

FOUR

The Sacral Chakra
or Svadisthana

If the Root chakra is the vehicle of the body, the Sacral chakra is its temple, and it is here that we explore our own needs and desires, initially through our five senses. It is also the seat of sexuality and reproduction, drawing primal energy from the Root chakra. It is the chakra of the Moon and of desire.

It has been called the place where death and procreation meet, for the body here, unlike the mortal physical body governed by the Root chakra, forms the first level of the Etheric or Spirit body. Some believe that this Spirit body is the part that survives death and is seen as a ghost by the living. You may sometimes find in meditation that you spontaneously move outside your Spirit body, though you may not be able to induce this state until you are more advanced in your chakra work.

The Sacral chakra is first activated at the pre-school stage when intuition and uninhibited imagination roam free. Many pre-school children are incredibly psychic. These intuitive qualities can be re-activated in adulthood as we work with this chakra.

Often called the wellspring of life, the Sacral chakra flows in an unregulated manner in children, veering between laughter and tears in seconds. This is the realm of emotions, of pure feeling, and it is from here that our humanity, empathy and ability to relate to others, to feel their joy or pain, emanate.

Control is usually imposed by the reasoning powers of the Solar Plexus chakra, rather than by external rules or a fear of punishment.

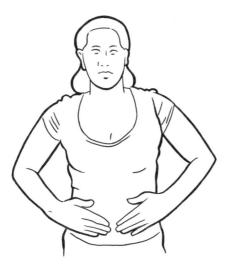

*Charging the
Sacral chakra*

Think of the three-year-old child, writhing, yelling on the floor, a pure bundle of wants, needs and desires as yet unformulated. 'Want never gets,' my mother informed me regularly throughout my formative years, because that was what she had learned. This can set up a cycle of guilt, a denial of needs and a projection of our own desires and needs on to others – we may even go on to marry that projection. What is more, in these formative years when innocent sensuality and embryo sexuality are manifest as a desire to explore the body and its sensations, we can receive the message that sex is dirty, especially if associated in the unconscious with over-rigorous bowel and bladder training.

This chakra tends to be fairly dormant during the pre-adolescent school years but burgeons again in adolescence as sexuality and emotions find a focus in a special person – our first true love. We then begin the eternal dance of self/other that is fully developed in identity issues in the higher Solar Plexus chakra.

Some of us have a lot of work to do to rekindle self-love and self-esteem and to rewrite a script in which our feelings were too often suppressed and our self-worth denied by adults who themselves were struggling at this chakra level.

Society especially is obsessed with the body beautiful and young, overemphasising the need for the approval of others and to conform to a stereotyped ideal to be of value and loved.

So many beautiful women are on a constant diet and see only their defects when they look in the mirror. We may need to re-learn that our desires and needs are not selfish and that we can recapture as adults the intuitive powers that can be our best guide to action if facts are conflicting or a situation uncertain.

Location of the Sacral chakra

This chakra is seated in the sacrum/lower abdomen, around the reproductive system and focuses on all aspects of physical comfort or satisfaction. It controls the blood, all bodily fluids and hormones, the reproductive system, kidneys, circulation and bladder and is a chakra especially sensitive to stress and imbalance if we get out of harmony with our natural cycles. Blockages can show themselves as fluid retention, menstrual or menopausal problems, mood swings, impotence in men and an inability in women to relax in sex. These can be manifest in both sexes as an overemphasis on sexual performance and flitting from one partner to another in a search for satisfaction.

Disorders involving physical indulgence to seek emotional satisfaction, especially eating disorders, smoking, and drug and alcohol abuse, can also result from blockages.

Sacral chakra correspondences

This information will help you to understand the correspondences related to the Sacral chakra.

Colour

Orange is the colour of the Sacral chakra.

This ritual uses the colour orange to strengthen the Sacral chakra.

- Light an orange candle and sit in your special place either by moonlight or at dawn or sunset as orange floods the sky.

- Visualise yourself breathing in orange light from the candle or from orange flowers that grow in your region. Gently exhale the darkness.

- At weekends, instead of using electricity, try to make the orange sunset and sunrise your marker points. In this way you will start to get in touch with your inner ebbs and flows.

- On these occasions when you live by natural light, light your orange candle at dusk and when it is burned through sit or lie quietly in the darkness until you fall asleep. Be sure to put the candle somewhere safe.

- Leave the curtains open so that you wake with the dawn. This is the rhythm our agricultural ancestors followed, but 24-hour-a-day lighting, heating, working and shopping has cut us off from the natural rhythms. (See also Tuning into Moon time on page 51 of this chapter.)

- You can also work with silver, the colour of the Moon goddesses who rule this chakra and who are especially related to the reproductive and sexual aspects of the chakra.

Element

Water is the element corresponding to the Sacral chakra.

This chakra is ruled by goddesses of the sea so the proximity of water and moonlight, which has strong associations with the sea, can make a powerful stimulus for freeing the energies.

- Spend time by the sea if you can, writing your wishes, desires and needs in the sand with a stick. Allow this stick to be taken by the sea at tide turn – its most powerful moment.

- Cast shells into the sea on to the seventh wave as the tide comes in, naming a wish for each one.

- Paddle into the sea and set dying petals afloat on the ebb tide, naming any guilt or inhibitions that you wish to be carried away.

- You can use any flowing water source if you cannot visit the ocean.

- Swim or paddle in the sea when the moonlight casts a pathway of light. Alternatively, improvise with a swimming pool lit by artificial lights that cast circles on the surface of the water.

- Swim in the light water and feel your Sacral energies flowing freely and all doubts about your worth flowing away.

- Make your own Sacral chakra water by half-filling a silver or glass bowl with spring water. Leave the bowl in the moonlight on the night of the Full Moon so that the water turns silver. If the Moon is not shining, leave it anyway, as it will absorb Moon energies. You can also light a ring of silver candles around the bowl.

- Use your chakra water in your bath. Sip your chakra water when you need the strengths of the Sacral chakra in your life or warm a little and massage it first anti-clockwise and then clockwise into your Sacral chakra to clear blockages and to increase self-esteem.

Symbol

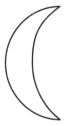

The crescent Moon in orange and silver is the symbol of the Sacral chakra.

Paint orange and silver crescents, cover them with glitter and hang them over your bed so that moonlight or silver candlelight shines on them as you meditate.

Even better, meditate on the silver crescent in the sky, breathing in the silver light and then closing your eyes, exhaling darkness. Establish a regular rhythm until you are filled with light.

Mantra sound

Vam is the mantra sound of the Sacral chakra.

Planet)〕

The Moon is the planet related to the Sacral chakra.

Though there are Moon gods, lunar energies are primarily yin/female/anima in men and women (see the deities listed below).

Throughout history and in many cultures, the Moon has been worshipped as a triple goddess, either as three sisters or daughter, mother and grandmother. Each of these represents a phase of lunar energy that is mirrored in the monthly cyclical increase and decline in energies and in the actual life cycle of both men and women as they increase in wisdom and maturity. The three phases of monthly energies start with the period of new beginnings and gently increasing energies that we can use to initiate projects and to improve any matter in our lives. Then is the brief period around the Full Moon when we have a sudden surge of energy in our lives. Since, at this time, the Sun is in direct opposition to the Moon astrologically, this can also be a period of instability and change. Finally comes the waning period when we can finish our month's projects and clear the decks for another month.

The Moon rules Cancer (22 June–22 July) and Sacral chakra work is especially potent during that period. Those born during this period generally find Sacral chakra work easiest.

Monday, the day of the Moon, is especially good for Sacral chakra work.

Archangel

Gabriel, Archangel of the Moon and the messenger, is associated with the Sacral chakra.

Gabriel offers compassion and acceptance of the weaknesses of self and others. He can be felt with each new Moon, especially on the day before the crescent is visible in the sky, also in places close to water. He brings self-love, diminishes self-destructive tendencies and replaces them with gentle growth of new hope and connection with others.

Light a silver candle and create or buy a tiny water feature with small pump, green plants, shells and Sacral chakra crystals. Allow Gabriel to speak to you in the sound of the water.

Deities

All Moon and Water goddesses and the Virgin Mary are related to the Sacral chakra.

The Virgin Mary, as Stella Maris (star of the sea), still protects sailors as they navigate across the oceans. In her blue robe covered in stars, she is often depicted with a crescent moon beneath her feet.

Selene is the Greek goddess specially associated with the Full Moon, sometimes forming a triplicity with Diana, the virgin huntress and Hecate, the crone who guides souls through the Underworld and protects sailors.

Twin sister of Helios the Sun god, Selene rises from the sea in her chariot drawn by white horses at night and rides high in the sky in her Full Moon.

She is invoked for fertility, at the time of the Full Moon, and by all who seek the power of intuition and inspiration.

Yemaya–Olokun, of the Yoruba peoples in West Africa, is an elemental force who not only lives in, but is the sea. Yemaya, also called Iemanja and the Womb of Creation, is the bringer of dreams and prosperity. In Brazil, on New Year's Eve, where she is worshipped by followers of Santeria, altars are created on the shore with candles and food that are accepted by Yemaya on the morning tide.

Drawing down the Moon goddess

In the Western magical tradition, the Full Moon is used as a focus to draw down cosmic energies personified by the Moon goddess. The ritual is often performed by a priestess, but men can also successfully channel higher energies from this force. This can be a good way of empowering the Sacral chakra, the home of lunar energies.

- When the Full Moon is bright in the sky, fill a large silver dish with spring water.

- Use a silver mirror to direct the reflection of the Moon into the water.

- Focus on the reflected lunar disc, and, as you breathe regularly, visualise the reflection and your Sacral chakra expanding together. Continue until the two have merged and you are completely enclosed in silver.

- Begin to speak (you may like to have a tape recorder close so you can play it back afterwards) as though you were talking to the goddess about your desires, your feelings and your needs. Do not pause to analyse what you are saying and keep talking even if your words do not seem to make sense to the logical side of your mind.

- When you are ready, allow the energies to fade and the Moon to recede, so that all you feel is the pulsating of your Sacral chakra and perhaps an aura of silver.

- Pour the water into the earth, or the soil in a plant pot if you are working indoors.

- Lie still in the moonlight and let dreams and images come and go.

- Immediately before you sleep, listen to the tape, but again do not analyse it.

- You may have significant dreams or may even feel that your spirit has temporarily left your body in sleep and wandered in strange but exciting lands.

- The next evening, if you listen to the tape while sitting by candlelight, you may find a thread running through the flow of words which will help to clarify any confused emotions you have and make you aware of unacknowledged needs.

Creatures

Fish, dolphins and all sea creatures are related to the Sacral chakra.

If you can, keep goldfish or another orange or silver species of fish in your home or outside. As you watch your fish moving, you can flow with them in underwater caverns and feel your own inner waters flowing freely and creatively. Add tiny chakra crystals to the water.

Crystals

Banded orange agate, amber, aquamarine, orange calcite, carnelian, coral, fluorite, moonstone and rutilated quartz correspond with the Sacral chakra.

Place a Sacral chakra crystal into an orange glass bottle and pour in some spring water. Leave the bottle open during daylight hours; then, at dusk, put the lid or a cork in the bottle. Pour some of the water into your bath, massaging around the Sacral chakra with the water and enjoying the sensation of your fingers on your skin.

You can also drink the water whenever you feel lacking in self-worth, unloved or unlovely.

Incenses and oils

Clary sage, jasmine, lotus, myrrh, rosewood and ylang-ylang relate to the Sacral chakra.

Use oils from this list to free blockages in the Sacral chakra, and bring harmony and healing.

- Light orange and silver candles around the bath.
- Add a few drops of Sacral essential oil to your bath water and, closing your eyes, allow the fragrance to enter your body.
- When you have finished, get out and dry yourself; then swirl the water nine times using the traditional chant:

Guilt and sorrow flow from me,

Leaving only harmony.

- Let all your self-doubt drain away with the water.

Herbs

Freesia, gardenia, lemon balm, lily, poppy and wintergreen are the herbs that correspond to and can help to stimulate the Sacral chakra.

- Tie them in a muslin bag or a pair of old tights and float them in the bath or secure them under the hot tap so that the water filters through them as you run the bath.

- Alternatively, make an infusion (a tea) of the herbs with boiling water, leave for five minutes, strain and add the liquid to the bath water.

See page 156 for herb books listing specific properties. If you are pregnant or suffer from medical conditions such as diabetes or high blood pressure, check that these herbs are safe by checking in a book on herbs or aromatherapy, or asking a pharmacist or herbalist. Some herbs and oils, for example clary sage, myrrh, poppy and wintergreen should not be used in pregnancy (see also page 123).

Trees

Alder, eucalyptus, lemon tree, willow and all trees that grow by water are associated with the Sacral chakra.

Intuition is one of the gifts that you can use when the chakra is functioning efficiently. Your intuitive awareness can be reawakened whether you are free to go outside or are restricted to working indoors.

- If possible, visit a Moon tree growing by water when the Moon is bright and the leaves are casting shadows in the water.

- If you are working indoors, hang a small bough of your chosen Moon tree over a bowl of water that is lit by silver candles. Take care when positioning the candles.

- Now ask a question and drop a pure white pebble into the water or a chakra crystal into your bowl. As the water ripples, gaze intently and say or write the first image that comes into your mind.

- Drop a second and third stone or crystal into the water and again record the images. You might find it easier to draw them.

- Reading the three images as a story, you will find that they answer your question.

- Note your images and your interpretation in alphabetical order in your chakra journal.

- You will find this personal symbol system increasingly useful as your psychic powers unfold through working with the higher chakras.

Affirmation

'I desire' is the affirmation for the Sacral chakra.

Working with the Sacral chakra

The close association of the Sacral chakra with the Moon is the key to harmonising this chakra. By learning to recognise the cycles of the Moon and to align our lives with these cycles, we can overcome much of the stress in our everyday lives.

The first calendars were usually based on the regular cycle of the Moon's waxing and waning. We know that the Moon governs the tides, and our own hormones seem to ebb and flow with the lunar cycle. In some of the few remaining indigenous societies, women still ovulate on the Full Moon and menstruate when the Moon is no longer visible in the sky at the end of the waning cycle and beginning of the new. Some women find that by reharmonising their cycles with the Moon, conception is easier. This is done by beginning the lunar month with gentle activity that increases slowly in pace, then working to peak power and action at the Full Moon and resting more and looking to their inner world during the waning Moon periods. Over a number of months the energies and the menstrual cycle move into harmony with the actual Moon cycle.

You will find that you become increasingly energetic and dynamic as the Moon increases in size. You may quarrel more but also make passionate love and make major leaps in inspiration at the Full Moon. As the Moon wanes, so you will feel less like frantic activity and need to pace yourself, cutting out non-essential activities and decisions at the end of the cycle.

It is the spirit's and body's way of telling you to slow down and regenerate. If we can do this, then problems such as irritability or PMT, themselves symptoms of a Sacral chakra out of harmony, will lessen dramatically.

Tuning into Moon time

The cycle from New Moon to New Moon lasts 29.5 days but because the Moon has an irregular orbit, its rising and setting times will vary each day by up to an hour. Newspapers and diaries usually give the daily rising and setting times.

For the first two or three days of the Moon cycle it is not visible in the sky; in this true new Moon phase all the energies are still hidden and so it is the time for plans and dreams. The ancients believed that the Moon was reborn when the crescent first appeared in the sky around the third day.

• Each day spend a few days looking at the sky. Use a sky globe or one of the excellent computer programmes that show where the Moon is in the sky, even if it is overcast.

- On clear nights you will see how it rises diagonally. You can use a tree or the roof of a house or even a tall fence to note the position at a specific time of the night and month. Next month it will be slightly different as a result of the irregular orbit. Don't be fooled in the waning phase. Later in the phase, you may see in the early morning yesterday's Moon not yet set.

- Each night note what the Moon makes you feel like doing – lighting a candle, making love, dancing in the garden, cleaning out a cupboard, having an argument or doing absolutely nothing.

- If you monitor these feelings for three or four months, you will find your own Moon pattern emerging and will begin to understand why you feel the way you do (seemingly irrationally sometimes). Most importantly, you will learn to maximise your best Moon times for action or for contemplation, for a trip to a theme park or a walk in the woods.

- During the waning period when you may feel more stressed and less energetic, try to make a quiet time every day even for a few minutes when you can light a silver candle and burn one of the oils or incenses of the Moon. Jasmine, lotus and myrrh are especially soothing for a Sacral chakra overburdened with the demands of others.

FIVE

The Solar Plexus Chakra or Manipura

This is the chakra of Fire and power. *Manipura* means precious gems. It is the highest of the three personal chakras (Root, Sacral and Solar Plexus), and many people who do not develop psychically operate quite successfully through these three in the everyday world and in their relationships.

Animals, it is believed, possess the two lower chakras, although others would argue that the loyalty and altruism shown by some domesticated pets would indicate that they may attain higher levels of awareness through love for a human.

The Solar Plexus chakra is concerned with conscious thought, rationalisation and directed will of all the Root energies and the emotions and driving force of desire in the Sacral chakra.

Blockages in this chakra and in the two lower ones can be caused by worry, swings of emotion, anger and negative feelings. Though the causes of these may be external, at this chakra level we can choose not to be angry, not to worry about what cannot be changed, not to dissipate our energies on living our lives through others or primarily to satisfy their needs.

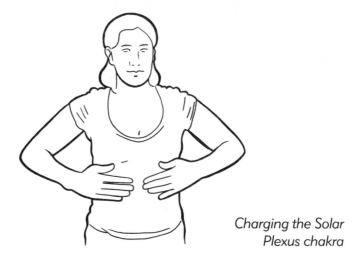

*Charging the Solar
Plexus chakra*

This then is an important chakra, for it is about making choices. Of course, merely deciding that we want improvements does not mean we can wave a magic wand over our finances, our career or our relationships. But we can rather than worrying, burying our heads in the sand or yelling, take steps to deal with even the most difficult situations or conversely accept that they cannot be changed.

As a result, this and the chakras below will unblock quite spontaneously as negativity is replaced by focus and planning and you learn to act rather than react.

You, as separate from others, your essential and unique self, thought as opposed to feeling manifest in the Sacral chakra or the instinctive aspects of the Root chakra, are the keys to this chakra. Of course, if you operated through this chakra alone, it would make you an arid, unimaginative person. There are times, however, when you may need the assertiveness and will power to reset your course or resist the pressures of others. But if you do draw energy from below, then you will attain the integration inherent in this chakra.

When people use expressions such as, 'I cannot stomach his/her view or way of life', they are using the image of the physical stomach processing and transforming the food source and eliminating waste matter. Physically, this chakra is centred on the digestive processes (see overleaf). It is, therefore, said to absorb the life force or *prana* from living food such as fruit, vegetables and seeds and to integrate both the forces of the lower chakras and the effects of the outside world and other people, rejecting what is redundant or not of use.

Location of the Solar Plexus chakra

The third chakra is to be found above the navel around the stomach area or in some systems further up towards the central cavity of the lungs. Confusion arises because some systems place another major chakra around this area, called the spleen, and in modern practice the two have been combined. The Solar Plexus chakra can therefore either be placed closer to the lower two, to which it belongs as the trio of personal chakras, or higher towards the Heart chakra. Either way, it rules the stomach and the digestion.

Hold a pendulum 2–3 cm (1 in) above this area and notice where you feel the pull and the swirling of the vortex in the centre. Use the pendulum's positive swing to identify the circumference of this chakra. (The positive swing is usually a clockwise circle or ellipse, but you can experiment by thinking of a happy event and seeing which way the pendulum moves in response to your thoughts.) Remember that because the chakras are part of the higher vibrational levels of the body, you may feel the central vortex at a distance from your body, according to how many chakra levels are operating efficiently. The seven levels of the aura extend an arm span to either side of the body, and far more than this as you become spiritually evolved, for the aura is in theory limitless and the highest level merges with cosmic energies. Indeed the aura of Gautama Buddha was said to extend several miles and so the chakras within him also radiated far and wide.

The function of the Solar Plexus chakra is to galvanise personal power and individuality and to integrate experience.

Its body parts include digestion, the liver, spleen, gall bladder, stomach and small intestine and the metabolism. Digestive disorders and hyperactivity can result from imbalances and blockages.

On a psychological level, a lack of self-confidence, obsessions, finding fault with others and an inability to empathise can result from the inefficient working of this chakra.

Activating this chakra involves lots of movement to kindle dormant energies and so I have included a number of rituals that you can adapt for the other chakras when you feel that energies are particularly sluggish.

Solar Plexus chakra correspondences

Colour

The colour of the Solar Plexus chakra is yellow.

The power of the Solar Plexus chakra colour can be captured in a wax talisman.

Making a wax talisman
- Light a small, broad, yellow beeswax candle on a metal tray or fireproof dish.
- Allow it to burn down and, as you look into the flame through half-closed eyes, allow images to come and go.
- When an image is disturbing or evokes anxiety, close your eyes and shrink it in your mind's vision until it becomes a dot in the candle flame and then disappears.
- If an image appears that makes you feel powerful, happy or confident again, close your eyes and let the image expand until it encloses you in pure yellow light and joy.
- When the wax is molten, carve in it with a knife or awl, a single word or symbol of power.
- Draw a circle in the molten wax around your power symbol and then draw a larger enclosing circle around the two, which you can cut out with a knife.
- Sprinkle a circle of salt, make a second circle in smoke with one of your Solar Plexus incenses (see page 61) and finally make a circle of pure spring water. As you do this, repeat the word or the name of the symbol you have inscribed over and over, faster and louder until you finish with a final shout and the words:

So shall it be.

- Wrap your talisman in a small piece of white silk and keep it always near you in a drawstring bag or purse.
- Replace it when it is cracked and bury the old talisman under one of your chakra trees.

Element

Fire is the element associated with the Solar Plexus chakra.

Fire is perhaps the most exciting element to work with in all its forms. Though the Sun is primarily associated with the Crown chakra, it is an important source of heat as well as light.

Walking in the sunshine, especially in sandy places, fills this chakra with natural power. Storms with lightning are also sources of natural fire power, as are sites of volcanic activity.

In the section on working with the Solar Plexus chakra, I write about kindling and working with the ancient ritual form of fire, the nyd fire. Whether you light huge, yellow candles in a dish or pot of sand, a bonfire or a small fire in a metal tray, move slowly around the source of heat and light at a safe distance, allowing your body to sway like the flames, so that you connect with the power of the fire.

- Light outdoor candles and torches or four large yellow or red candles in floor holders indoors to make a circle of fire.

- Move inside your fire circle, perhaps waving yellow and red ribbons or small scarves. Move with rhythm, but be careful not to catch the flames.

- You might like to play drum music to establish the rhythm.

- As you dance, chant:

> *Fire of power, power of fire,*
>
> *Flames that rise ever higher,*
>
> *Power to attain my heart's desire.*

- Again chant faster and end with a final leap, throwing your arms in the air, calling:

> *I am pure fire.*

Symbol

A yellow inverted triangle is the symbol of the Solar Plexus chakra.

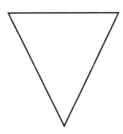

You can make this symbol even more powerful by writing your name within the triangle, beginning with the last letter at the bottom so that your power increases. Below I have illustrated this idea with my name, Cassandra:

CASSANDRA

ASSANDRA

SSANDRA

SANDRA

ANDRA

NDRA

DRA

RA

A

If you have a short name, add your middle or surname. Recite it as you write.

Mantra sound

Rum (pronounced R-ooo-m) is the mantra sound of the Solar Plexus chakra.

Planet ♂

Mars is the planet of the Solar Plexus chakra.

The Roman warrior god, Mars, was legendary father of Romulus and Remus, the founders of Rome. As god of both agriculture and war, he represented the ideal Roman, first as a farmer and then as a conqueror. The agricultural fire festivals are therefore linked with his power. He corresponds mythologically with the Greek Ares and Tiw or Tyr, the Viking altruistic warrior god who sacrificed his sword arm to save the other deities – and gave his name to Tuesday.

Mars rules Aries (21 March–20 April) and is the co-ruler of Scorpio (24 October–22 November). Solar Plexus chakra work is especially potent during these periods and on Tuesdays. Those born during these times will generally find Solar Plexus chakra work easiest.

You can use the courage of Mars to cut through fear, anger and anxiety by drawing or writing on paper the inner monster you most fear and scribbling negative feelings all over it. Then cut it up with sharp scissors (iron and steel are the metals of Mars) and throw the scraps away or burn them.

Archangel

Samael, angel of the Solar Plexus chakra, is the Archangel who rules the planet Mars and Tuesday.

He is sometimes called the Severity of God and as such is an angel of cleansing and of righteous anger.

Samael the avenger, offers protection to the weak and vulnerable, and cleanses doubts and weakness, replacing them with spiritual courage to stand against what is corrupt, especially those who abuse power.

He is a good focus if invoked in a dark red or burgundy candle and will offer wisdom not only on issues of personal fears and anger, but on ways of directing power towards helping to right environmental and more global injustices (more of this in the next chapter).

Deities

Brighid, Agni, goddesses and gods of fire relate to the Solar Plexus chakra.

The Celtic Brighid was once a Sun goddess, born, according to legend, at sunrise. As she entered the world a shaft of fire blazed from her head linking earth with heaven.

The holy fire at the saint's shrine in Kildare, dedicated originally to the goddess and then to Saint Bridget in the Christian tradition, is believed to have burned unquenched for more than a thousand years. It was tended first by 19 virgin priestesses called the Daughters of the Sacred Flame and later by the nuns of the Abbey at Kildare.

In both cases, the goddess and later the saint were said to care for the fire on the twentieth day of the cycle.

In India, the great Fire god was Agni, sometimes regarded as an aspect of the Sun god. He ruled not only over the fires of lightning and heaven but the sacred fires on Earth as well. Agni carried sacrifices from man to the gods on the dark canopy of smoke from the sacrificial fires on Earth.

In ancient Mexico, Xiuhtecutli, the Fire god, was also the god of the domestic hearth. Every morning and evening, Mexican families offered him food and drink. His body was flame-coloured and a yellow serpent rested over his back to represent the flickering flames.

Creating a sacred hearth

Throughout the world and for thousands of years the sacred hearth has formed the centre of the home. Indeed the Latin word for the domestic hearth was *focus*.

Here it was believed living members of the family could gather for food and warmth and so too the wise ancestors might draw near (see the Heart chakra).

In a number of cultures in both eastern and western Europe and Mediterranean lands and in those places in the New World where their descendants settled, a small part of the family meal would be placed on the fire as an offering to the deities and spirits of Fire.

- If you have an open fire, sprinkle on to the coals Solar Plexus herbs (for example allspice or basil, see page 61) or indeed herbs of any other chakra that needs strengthening.

- If the fireplace is empty, fill it with red and yellow flowers or branches from the Solar Plexus trees and, in the evening, light a yellow candle and sit quietly, absorbing the energies.

- A large iron pot as a focal point (the original witches' cauldrons were in fact cooking pots) can serve the same purpose.

Creatures

The ram, salamander and phoenix are creatures of the Solar Plexus chakra.

According to Greek myth, the ram, the animal of Aries, was covered with the fabled golden fleece, as sought by Jason and the Argonauts.

The elemental creature of Fire, used in alchemy, is the salamander, the mythical lizard that lives within Fire (though the name is now given to a species of amphibious newts).

The most fabulous of the Fire creatures is the legendary phoenix. Of Arabian origin, the phoenix can also be found in the tales of many lands. In ancient Egypt it was the bird of the Sun god Ra and a sign of resurrection, as the sun was seen to be reborn with each new day.

The phoenix burned itself on a funeral pyre every five hundred years and a young phoenix rose golden from the ashes.

To the Chinese, the phoenix is one of the sacred creatures like the dragon, and in China and Japan its appearance foretold the coming of a great emperor or sage; images of the phoenix were carried or worn to ensure long life and health.

In the Western world, the phoenix was adopted by mediaeval alchemists and the resurrected glorious phoenix was the symbol of alchemy's ultimate aim of turning base metal into gold. The bird is described as having brilliant gold, red and purple feathers and being the size of a huge eagle.

- Burn two or three sticks of one of the Solar Plexus incenses in a vase or on a metal tray so you can collect the ashes.
- In traditional manner, bury some, cast some in flowing water and scatter the rest to the winds, calling out a message of power or determination that will be amplified by the energies.

Crystals

Golden beryl, yellow calcite, citrine, desert rose, tiger's eye and topaz are crystals that can be used to harmonise the Solar Plexus chakra.

- Make your Solar Plexus crystals more powerful by leaving them in a brass or gold-coloured dish filled with spring water from dawn until the Sun has reached its height at midday.
- The day of the summer solstice is particularly powerful, as are solar eclipses, even partial ones.
- Keep the water in a glass bottle to add to your bath or to massage on to your Solar Plexus if you feel afraid or over-emotional.

Incenses and oils

Cinnamon, copal, dragon's blood, juniper, lemon, pine and rosemary correspond to the Solar Plexus chakra.

- Use a large, firm incense stick that will not crumble. The outdoor kind is excellent for working in the open air. Light it in sunlight so the smoke becomes golden.
- Make nine circles of smoke clockwise around yourself, again focusing on a word or phrase that expresses self-confidence and courage – you could weave the affirmation (page 62) into a chant.
- Whenever you feel afraid, visualise your nine circles of power.

Herbs

Allspice, basil, coriander, ginger, peppermint and tarragon relate to the Solar Plexus chakra.

- Light a yellow candle in a broad-based holder.
- Place next to it a small dish of Solar Plexus herbs. Rosemary is best as it enhances mental acuity and focus. Rosemary is listed under Incenses and oils, all of which have basic herbal forms and so are interchangeable with the herb list. Rosemary, like juniper, is especially powerful since both are also Crown chakra herbs.
- Take a grain or two at a time and burn them in the candle flame.

- As you do so, name your strengths and talents, including those you have not yet developed and then say for each:

    This I will do, before the week/month/year is through.

- Create a realistic time frame for your affirmations in your chakra journal. You may allocate anything from two days for an urgent matter such as unanswered correspondence to ten years for a major life change, such as retiring to live in the sun.

- When you have finished, sit as the candle burns down and list the steps you need to take to fulfil each affirmation.

Trees

Hawthorn, holly, palm, pine and rowan are associated with the Solar Plexus chakra.

- Beneath one of the Solar Plexus trees or any large palm-type pot plant in the home, bury nuts to represent any fears or worries you have that are keeping you awake at night and blighting the pleasures of the day.

- Use large nuts for major worries.

- In time the shoots of an embryo tree may grow. Even if they do not, you have planted a symbol of new life. Make plans, however small, towards positive resolution or accepting what cannot be changed.

- When you feel a worry coming on, place a nut in a covered jar to contain the anxiety until you have time to bury it.

Affirmation

'I will' is the affirmation of the Solar Plexus chakra.

Working with the Solar Plexus chakra

Nyd, or need, fires, the central holy fires of the Teutonic and Celtic peoples, were kindled throughout the year. The first were at the early Spring festival of Brigantia (Christianised as Candlemas at the beginning of February), then at Spring Equinox around 21 March (later Easter), at Beltane or May Eve at the end of April, at the Summer Solstice or Midsummer around 21 June, at the First Corn Harvest, Lughnassadh or Lammas at the beginning of August, at the Autumn Equinox or Harvest Home around 23 September, at Samhain or Hallowe'en on 31 October to welcome the ancestors home and finally at the Midwinter Solstice or Christmas around 21 December (the rebirth of light and the Sun or the Son of God).

The fire was kindled with nine different kinds of wood: alder, ash, birch, elm, hazel, hawthorn, oak, rowan and willow. Sticks were rubbed together or a more elaborate oaken spindle was turned in an oaken log-socket, from which all other fires were lit.

Though it is called a nyd or need fire, the purpose is to fulfil one's own needs, rather than always looking to others, using one's inner flame and inspiration. Hence the fires were kindled by friction.

- Light a fire – even a few sticks in a metal dish will serve, but a bonfire is preferable. You can use any of the sacred woods or ones that are indigenous to your region.

- Unless you are versed in woodcraft, you may need to light your fire by more conventional means, but as you do so, visualise the flame of inspiration and power within your Solar Plexus being kindled.

- Carefully place a longer branch (or twig, in the case of a smaller fire) in the flame so it begins to smoulder. Then circle the fire with it three times, before casting it into the centre of the flames, saying:

Fire increase and multiply, power in me intensify

From the Earth to the sky.

- Light as many twigs or branches as you wish until you are filled with joy and inspiration. If you can work close to one of the old festivals, the experience will be even more significant. This will help to strengthen your Sacral chakra work. You can also light fires on the Full Moon.

SIX

The Heart Chakra
or Anahata

This is the chakra of the winds and of love. It forms a transition between the three personal chakras and those that connect with the universal energy field. Like any transitional point, it relates both to personal and more global levels of functioning.

This chakra is activated in love relationships between permanent partners and family members and is associated with fidelity and spiritual love, for example the mother who will risk her life for a child, or a man or woman who nurses an ageing or disabled relative willingly.

More generally it increases our capacity for harmony and inner peace that relieves us of the see-saw of the Sacral chakra mood swings. This still core can offer protection against external negativity and enable us to act rather than react (see pages 75 and 106 for centring and stilling exercises).

It strengthens an awareness of our interconnectedness with all life, whether animal, bird, crystal or plant. In societies where the written word was less important than orally transmitted wisdom, for example Celtic Druidry, Australian Aboriginal spirituality or Native American wisdom, this chakra was one of the personal energy centres through which ordinary men and women experienced these higher levels of awareness in their everyday lives.

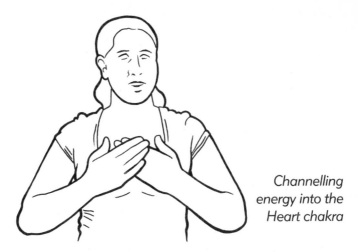

*Channelling
energy into the
Heart chakra*

Through this chakra comes also knowledge and, if we wish for it, direct experience of higher planes of beings, especially devas and wise nature spirits that co-exist alongside our world but at a higher vibrational level. This chakra enables us to reach the level of existence that resonates with the astral level of our Spirit body, which in turn corresponds to the substance of these higher beings (see page 21).

The Heart chakra rules the all-important minor chakras in the palm of each hand and so is a source of healing power, especially when amplified by crystals, herbs and other natural forces. However, you may as you work with this chakra find that you are able to channel the pure life force from the cosmos (see page 127). This higher healing energy is channelled from the universe, via the Crown, Brow and Throat chakras, circulates through the Heart chakra (see diagram), and out through the fingers. As a gateway chakra it can draw energies from the higher as well as the lower chakras (see page 128 for details of using chakra healing).

The Heart chakra is said to be the seat of the soul and the point at which we are truly aware of our spiritual potential and connection with the higher dimensions. When this chakra is fully developed, we can see or sense the presence of what are called ghosts in modern westernised culture, but which other, older cultures call the wise ancestors, whose guidance may appear through signs or through a strong connection with our heritage (see page 99 for past life work).

Location of the Heart chakra

The Heart chakra is situated in the centre of the chest, radiating over heart, lungs, breasts and also hands and arms. Compassion and transformation of our everyday lives through connection with our still centre of being are results of a clear Heart chakra. Constant coughs, breathing difficulties and allergies can be a result of blockage or imbalance, as can oversensitivity to the problems of others that leaves us anxious but unable to offer real help.

Heart chakra correspondences

Colour

Green and pink are associated with the Heart chakra.

The most powerful form of colour is that found in living plants and flowers, as you can absorb the life force by visualising the green light that comes from them and gently inhaling this through your nose as you breathe, while picturing it spreading through your whole body. The mediaeval mystic Hildegard von Bingen called this process the greening principle or *veriditas*.

- Fill your work space with greenery and keep pink flowers in your special place while you are working with the energies of this chakra. Put moss agate or jade in the soil or water to keep them fresh.

- When you feel tired or stressed, create a Druidic grove by making a circle of tall pot plants or sit in an actual grove of bushes and trees (see page 74 for the list of chakra trees).

- Visualise shafts of pure green light emanating from each, forming the spokes of a wheel in whose hub you are sitting.

- Gently inhale first for a count of one and then exhale, then for a count of two and exhale for two, increasing to a level at which you are comfortable.

- Feel the light entering through your Heart chakra and circulating up and downwards through every nadir or psychic channel and spiralling, purifying and gently healing any pain, tension and unravelling blockages and filtering any darkness into the ground through your feet.

Element

The element associated with the Heart chakra is Air.

The four winds are central to Heart chakra work, as a means of allowing the life force to open channels that have become clogged and spring clean your entire chakra system, but especially the Heart.

Stand on top of a high hill on a windy day or in the middle of a windy plain. Open your arms wide and spin around, with long trailing scarves around your neck and in each hand. As you did when you were a child, shout all the things you would like to say if you dared or were able, but which you hold in your heart (more of this in the next chapter).

Fly feathers, or send kites and balloons high into the air, tying to the string luggage tags or streamers of paper on which you have written ways in which you wish to free your life of stagnation or attachments to destructive people or situations.

Afterwards run down the hill or walk with your arms high and allow the wind to carry you in your mind's vision to where you would most like to be.

Symbol

The six-pointed star is the symbol of the Heart chakra.

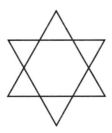

This star is known as Solomon's seal after the wise king in the Bible, symbol of total balance. The two triangles of the seal are the triangle of the alchemical and magical symbol for the Water element descending and the triangle of Fire ascending. With the mingling of these elements are also formed the triangles of Air and Earth. The triangles of the four elements (Earth, Air, Fire and Water) fuse into the middle quintessential shape of the pentagram (five points). The six external points of the star and its centre give the magical seven spaces, seven being a sacred number of perfection.

Practise drawing this symbol without taking your pen off the paper, over and over again to form a pattern. Then, if you wish, colour the individual spaces to form a mosaic and use the pattern in meditation. Sometimes the symbol is coloured all in green.

Mantra sound

Yam is the mantra sound associated with the Heart chakra.

Planet ♀

Venus is the planet of the Heart chakra.

Venus is traditionally associated with love and passion. However, Venus was, like her Greek counterpart, Aphrodite (see Deities, page 69) originally a goddess of time and fate and a virgin in the sense that she belonged to no man. Venus rules harmony and peace, beauty, the arts, crafts and music, relationships and the slow but sure growth of prosperity, for Venus rules all matters of growth. Like the Moon she can be invoked for horticulture and the environment.

All these are qualities reflected in a well-functioning Heart chakra.

Venus is sometimes known as the Morning or Evening Star and at her brightest she is the most brilliant object in the sky besides the Sun and Moon.

Use a sky globe or computer program to locate Venus in the sky in the morning or evening and stand quietly, feeling the Heart chakra centre opening to receive the brilliant light, breathing in the harmony and beauty and exhaling all that is ugly or disharmonious as grey mist.

Venus rules Taurus (21 April–21 May) and Libra (23 September–23 October). Heart chakra work is especially potent during these Sun sign periods and every Friday, the day of Venus. Those born during these times generally find Heart chakra work easiest.

Archangel

Anael, the angel of the Heart chakra, is the Archangel who rules over Venus and Friday. He is also the regenerator, one of the seven angels of creation, the Prince of Archangels, and he controls kings and kingdoms.

His is pure altruistic love – love of one's fellow beings and of all creatures in the universe. He can be invoked for all matters of forgiveness both to ourselves for what is past and to others that we may be free from their thrall.

Anael brings harmony to places and people and the restoration of natural balance, healing rainforests, bringing wildlife habitats to the city and greenery everywhere.

His fertility is that of the whole earth, rich in fruit, flowers, people and creatures of all kinds, whether living in the wild or in sanctuaries.

Use him to channel wisdom via natural sources such as the wind rustling in the trees. Botanical gardens are especially good just after opening time or before closing, as there are usually banks of flowers where you can sit for a while undisturbed and hear the voice of Anael on the soft breeze or see a face forming in the flowers.

You can contact devas, higher nature spirits in a similar manner (see Heart chakra crystals, page 72).

Deities

The love goddesses correspond with the Heart chakra.

The love goddesses are found in almost every age and culture. Like Venus, the Roman archetypal goddess of love, they were frequently not gentle creatures or seductresses concerned merely with attracting love and admiration. In their original forms they were feisty deities who were concerned with fate, with fertility and all kinds of abundance. Because they were linked with the growth cycle, they were also goddesses of decay and death.

The Heart chakra is a very strong one and, if you have compassion, then you will feel pain and become aware of suffering and issues of mortality. In her Evening Star aspect, Venus takes on a warrior and death goddess aspect, causing the snuffing out of the life force and all desire.

They also rule ritual or sacred sexuality. Aphrodite, Greek goddess of love, was originally an ancient Asian triple goddess of nature and her high priestess had ritual sex annually with the lord of the land as a way of renewing his sacred bargain to care for the earth and its people. This sacred marriage signifying the union of Earth and sky through sacred sex is found in many cultures.

In Hindu spirituality, Parvati, wife of Shiva, the Father god, was the beautiful young goddess of the mountains, a catalyst and power source without which Shiva would be impotent.

The marriage of Shiva and Parvati is still a model for humans, the great god and his Shakti or female essence, as the sacred marriage between Earth and Sky, the union between the lingam (a pillar representing the penis) and yoni (the representation in stone, wood or crystal of a vagina). They demonstrate the heights to be strived for by every married couple, momentarily experienced in tantric or sacred sexuality.

This chakra is one where sacred sexuality (see Chapter Twelve) can be used as a means of striving towards unity not only with a human partner, but through that union with all nature and ultimately to merge with cosmic bliss.

There are many ways of channelling this higher love and capacity in relationships with a significant other, both through the cosmic bliss attained through orgasm and in everyday life. Others channel this higher love into caring for sick or disabled people whether relations, friends or strangers or in working towards saving a rainforest, a threatened species or a war-torn land.

Find small ways of channelling this higher love into action, perhaps by joining an environmental group or making your own home and garden a place of harmony and beauty.

Creatures

The white dove and all birds are associated with the Heart chakra.

A far more powerful totem than it superficially appears, the dove features in the flood stories of the Babylonians, Hebrews, Chaldeans and Greeks, as a symbol of peace and reconciliation. It is an emblem of Venus, representing faithful and committed love. The dove is also sacred to the wise Greek goddess Athene and the symbol of Sophia, goddess of wisdom. In many cultures it is a female form of the Holy Spirit. It is, above all, the symbol of the Virgin Mary who sacrificed two turtledoves in the temple at her purification 40 days after the birth of Jesus.

The cooing of sacred pigeons or doves in the oracular groves dedicated to Zeus at Dodona were used for prophecy by the priestesses.

Finding a power bird

Spend time watching and feeding birds that are indigenous to your region and you will discover how each have special qualities. I have found that the birds that come to feed outside my caravan: song thrushes, blackbirds, chaffinches, starlings and jackdaws, have displayed distinct personalities, from the tap-dancing jackdaw thundering on my roof, to the two blackbirds, my personal power icons that wait on the doorstep if I go out.

One may become particularly friendly and he or she can, in the tradition of many lands, become your power bird, offering you particular strengths and qualities and resonating with your own true nature. As the Heart and the higher chakras become more active so you will find this communication becomes even more spiritual. The Native North Americans sought wisdom from the Clan Father and Mother of different animals and birds and Druids believed that it was possible to shapeshift or become spiritually one of the creatures with whom you resonated.

Visit also bird sanctuaries and parks where they can move freely and are not in cages and you may find that you feel an affinity to a more exotic creature.

Below I have listed a number of birds and their characteristics taken from mythology as well as personal observation.

By using a talisman, for example a feather, a picture or tiny representation of your power creature, you can invoke its strength at any time you need it.

Blackbird: Persistence.

Chaffinch: Courage in face of foes.

Cockerel: Protection.

Crane: Longevity and health.

Crow: Change and transformation.

Dove or pigeon: Reconciliation and love.

Duck: Prosperity.

Eagle: Nobility and vision.

Falcon or kestrel: Focus.

Flamingo: Grace.

Goose: Domestic happiness.

Hawk: Enlightenment.

Ibis: Unconscious and deep wisdom.

Ostrich: Justice.

Owl: Knowledge and conscious wisdom.

Parrot: Communication.

Peacock: Lasting happiness.

Pelican: Nurturing powers.

Raven: Hidden potential.

Seagull: Wide horizons.

Song thrush: Cheerfulness, even in adversity.

Stork: Fertility.

Swan (black): Female wisdom.

Swan (white): Creativity and magic.

Turkey: Abundance and altruism.

Crystals

Moss agate, aventurine, green calcite, emerald, jade, kunzite, rose quartz and green tourmaline are all crystals that correspond to the Heart chakra.

Since crystals are living essences with powerful auric fields, these Heart chakra crystals are a powerful way of contacting the higher nature spirits, especially the devas.

- Work outdoors, if possible where sunlight is filtering through trees, casting a green light.

- Make a circle around yourself of small chakra crystals.

- Sit on the earth or grass in the centre, holding a large chunk of unpolished rose quartz that is easy to obtain and inexpensive. Unpolished green calcite is also good for working with higher nature spirits.

- You are going to rely primarily on touch, so close your eyes and allow the sounds of nature, especially bird song, to fill your thoughts.

- Run your fingers over the surface of the crystal and allow impressions to form of a wise, green spirit, like an angel whose pink and green light is expanding to form a sphere around you.

- Open your eyes and, still holding the crystal, sit within the green and pink light and allow your deva to speak, perhaps of environmental concerns or of special places and ways you can attain the peace and stillness within your heart. Because this is a transition chakra, global and personal issues will mingle.

- Allow the green that represents growth and fertility and the pure pink of love to flow within you. Experience, through the devic power, pure love for humankind and all creatures and the interconnectedness between you and all creation.

Incenses and oils

Geranium, hyacinth, lilac, rose, strawberry, vanilla and vervain relate to the Heart chakra.

This chakra is the first level at which we can experience knowledge of the wise ancestors. This may be our own deceased grandparents, someone in the family hundreds of years before with whom we share an affinity or an ancestor from our root race many years ago, a Celt, a Viking, an ancient Egyptian or someone from the frozen North.

Honouring the wise ancestors

- Ideally you should carry out this ceremony at around midnight.
- Light five incense sticks in at least two of the chakra fragrances and set them in a circle around you.
- Sit close to an open window and place a clove of garlic on the window ledge, saying:

Welcome all who come in love and peace.

- Our ancestors, especially those in Celtic and Eastern European lands, believed that garlic offered protection against supernatural malevolence, and would place garlic on window sills to keep out evil spirits. The good dead could still enter.
- If there is a particular, deceased relation you would like to contact, use their favourite perfume or a memento.
- You will not see, nor would you necessarily welcome, a full-blown visitation, but you may sense a stirring in the air, a light touch like gossamer.
- You will sense a presence and, without words, will understand the purpose of the contact and the positive inflow of love into your heart from past generations. You may sense more than one person.
- When you are ready, thank the ancestor/s in your own words and say:

Go in peace.

- Sprinkle salt and water on the window ledge and door entrance, saying:

May only love remain and blessings.

- Close the window and bury the garlic outdoors or in a plant pot.

Herbs

Echinacea, feverfew, heather, mugwort, pennyroyal, thyme, verbena and yarrow are the herbs of the Heart chakra.

In order to work with the Heart chakra, it may be useful to have a number of the appropriate herbs conveniently to hand.

Making a Heart chakra herb garden

Plant Heart chakra herbs either in a patch in your garden or in window boxes or balcony tubs if you do not have a garden. Alternatively choose any flowers or herbs that you associate with love and harmony that are indigenous to your region (see page 156 for books on herbs that give other Heart chakra herbs that are ruled by Venus).

- Herbs should be planted one or two nights before the Full Moon.

- Add moss agate or jade crystals to the soil and water with crystal water in which Heart chakra crystals have been soaked for eight hours.

- When they are grown, cut the herbs on the day after the Full Moon.

- You can dry your herbs naturally and then put a few in a tiny, green, cloth sachet, fragranced with one of the Heart chakra essential oils and a tiny rose quartz.

- Keep this sachet pinned inside your clothes or in a breast pocket in a coat as close to the heart as possible. Alternatively carry it with you and sleep with it under your pillow. This will keep the Heart chakra functioning. Replace the sachet when it loses its fragrance.

Trees

Almond, apple, birch, cherry, olive and peach are the trees related to the Heart chakra.

- From fallen branches of your chosen tree or that of any fruit or flowering tree that is sacred to Venus, cut 20 small staves or use twigs of a similar size.

- On one side of each, scratch the bark and etch, draw or paint a symbol to represent the affirmative, the glyph of Venus or the six-pointed star.

- When you have a decision to make, sit quietly and perfectly still for five minutes close to a tree, holding all your twigs.

- Formulate a question relating to an issue close to your heart and silence all other questions or thoughts. The question should involve affirmative/negative answers, whether yes or no, go or stay, speak or be silent, act or wait.

- When you are ready, whisper the question and see it carried by the breeze.

- Cast your staves on the ground.

- Count the number of sticks on which the symbol is face uppermost. This will give you the answer that comes from your heart and is what you really want or what you know deep down.

- This method is invariably accurate for attuning you to the wisdom of this chakra that stands at the doorway between conscious and unconscious wisdom and so can spontaneously access both once we clear the space in our hearts.

- Do not be tempted to cast again. The more you trust your heart, which is very different from being swayed by emotion or sentimentality, the easier it becomes to connect with your inner well of wise and compassionate knowledge that is your best guide to right action.

Affirmation

'I embrace' is the affirmation corresponding to the Heart chakra.

Working with the Heart chakra

Centring is the logical progression that follows on from grounding (see page 41 in the Root chakra). It is very effective if you are receiving impressions from many different sources, you have conflicting demands on your time and energies or you feel that you are being drained of energy.

Sometimes you cannot shield yourself from the demands of others as you need to give out loving energies. You do, however, need to centre yourself, so that you do not become so sympathetic or concerned that your own peace of mind and ability to cope is destroyed.

- If you are centred, you are focused and you can concentrate or simply switch off from external pressures and allow your natural restorative energies to come into operation. I used to work on centring through the Brow or Third Eye chakra, but recently have discovered that the Heart chakra can act as a natural filter. Since it is connected so strongly to the minor chakras in the palm of the hand, this also forms a better channel.

- Hold your arms by your side and point your fingers downwards. If possible, stand on soil, sand or grass to make the direct connection with nature.

- Visualise all the energies that are not yours leaving your body, flowing downwards and out through the fingers into the Earth where they will be transformed into new, separate life.

- Shake your fingers and plunge them into water in which Heart chakra crystals have been soaked for eight hours.

- Then, using your hands with fingertips extended, make an arc all around your body, stooping to complete it around the feet. See the energies pouring into your fingers as pure pink light. Feel it rising up your arms, then returning to the Heart chakra.

- Carry this out weekly and then sit quietly, if possible in the open air, allowing your mind to become still and filled with green and pink spiralling energy.

SEVEN

The Throat Chakra
or Vishuddha

This is the chakra of purity and of time and space, which can suddenly expand your world view beyond the parameters of the material world into eternity and infinity.

Developing the chakras is like climbing to the top of a very tall cathedral. When you have walked up endless flights of dark steps with glimpses through slit windows, suddenly you emerge into the open air on to a narrow, circular balcony, and you can see all around. You know that you are not at the top, although for many people this view and height is quite enough in life as well as in cathedral towers. But if you want to go to the top and see the full vista you will need to carry on climbing up more even narrower steps. This is the level of the Throat chakra – so near to the top yet there is still a long way to go.

The Throat chakra, when developed, has been described as the vehicle for speaking the truth that is in your heart and for communication that is on a higher level. Power struggles, pettiness and the approval of others are superseded by wise, measured words where the compassion of the Heart is united with higher mental faculties and can draw cosmic wisdom from the two chakras above.

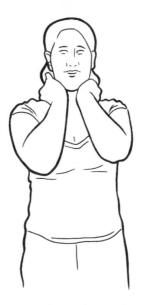

Charging the
Throat chakra

In gurus, spiritual teachers and prophets, the Throat chakra is highly evolved and as you work with it you may find that you too speak wise words that you did not realise were within you and also find yourself prophesying with accuracy about global as well as personal events.

In a practical sense, this is the chakra of pure creativity, as emotions and thoughts are synthesised and given expression in art, poetry, writing, music, dance, sacred architecture and, above all, in the way we live our lives, whether in high finance, bringing up children or just being, for the greatest good and by the highest ideals. It is where the unconscious and conscious synthesise so that we are not driven by impulses or drives, but can make choices because we are suddenly aware of the wider picture.

Because it is a higher chakra, the dream plane becomes more accessible as a source of wisdom. Astral travel or out-of-body travel that may have occurred spontaneously in the lower chakras, now becomes a means by which we can undergo shamanic journeys to explore other realms in dreams and during meditation, while working with a simple mandala for example (see page 87).

Because of the relation to inner and well as external sound, clairaudient abilities develop also as this chakra becomes activated, so that we can hear sounds from other dimensions and communicate wordlessly from mind to mind using telepathy. It is also the chakra of sacred form and working with sacred geometrical forms, such as labyrinths and circles, although here I concentrate on the mandala (see page 156 for books on other forms of sacred geometry).

Location of the Throat chakra

The Throat chakra is situated close to the Adam's apple in the centre of the neck. As well as the throat and speech organs, the Throat chakra controls the mouth, the neck and shoulders and the passages that run up to the ears. Blockages can be manifested as sore throats, swollen glands in the neck, mouth ulcers and ear problems. On a psychological level, confusion and incoherence result if the chakra is not working efficiently.

Throat chakra correspondences

Colour

Blue, the sky blue of summer sunshine, is the colour of the Throat chakra.

The best way to fill your Throat chakra with this blue light is to go outdoors in the summer sunshine, open your throat and sing at the top of your voice, any joyous song from any tradition or one you create as you go along, as you did when you were a child. Open your arms and dance, not a slow measure as you did for the Root chakra, but again with the uninhibited joy of childhood.

If the day is dull, put on bright blue scarves or drape yourself in sky blue cloth or even blue crepe paper, and sing to invoke the brightness. You may be rewarded by a patch in the clouds, which, as my late mother used to say, if big enough to make a sailor a pair of trousers, heralded a fine day after all.

Element

The element associated with the Throat chakra is sound, or in some systems ether itself, the synthesis of the other four elements.

Traditionally, sound was regarded as sacred, and music as a microcosm of the order of the universe, reflecting the harmonious movement of the heavenly bodies. Through it was seen the way to the ultimate, perfect silence at the heart of sound and of the cosmos. This is the archetypal sound of which all earthly chants and songs were a reflection.

Working with telepathy

Telepathy is silent communication between two people's minds – even if they are a great distance apart. It works best with someone with whom you have a loving connection. Though telepathy usually occurs quite spontaneously in families, working on developing telepathic communication will help to fine-tune the Throat chakra.

- Work with an absent friend or family member with whom you have regular contact.

- Pre-arrange a time, evening or morning, on two consecutive days when you will be undisturbed. When you first wake and just before you go to sleep are both times when conscious barriers are at their lowest.

- At first you may wish to focus on a pre-arranged topic, for example holidays you have shared.

- Address the person in your mind as though he or she were present.

- Because symbolism becomes an important channel of communication in this chakra and is a way in which much psychic information is processed and transmitted in the higher chakras, draw a symbol to represent the salient feature.

- As you do so, visualise the scene and recall any special phrases or names associated with it.

- At the same time the absent person should be sitting quietly listening and focusing on your message. He or she should write down any words or draw any images and symbols received.

- After the session you should both post the information to the other person.

- The next day, reverse roles and repeat. Continue this practice weekly.

- If you find it difficult, hold the actual symbol whose image you are transmitting, repeating its name in your head over and over.

- When comparing notes, you may find that you were transmitting related symbols to the experience, for example, if you were sending information about a friend who had a distinctive yellow car, your recipient might have drawn a symbol of a dog. This might not make sense until you recalled that together you had bought a toy dog to put on the parcel shelf for a joke.

Symbol

An inverted triangle surrounded by a circle is the symbol of the Throat chakra.

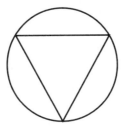

Add this design to your mandala pattern (see page 87). Colour it blue.

Mantra sound

Ham is the mantra sound associated with the Throat chakra.

Buddhists believe that if you meditate silently on mantras, either forming the words with your mouth without sounding them or repeating them in your mind, it forms a path to altered states of consciousness. In these states, it is possible for an adept ultimately to connect with his or her own divine nature, the source of divinity or, in Buddhist belief, Nirvana or cosmic bliss.

As sound is one of the key concepts of this chakra, you may like to create your own mantra, centred around some of the associations with this chakra, for example:

Sky of blue, speak true,

Ganesha renew.

You can, as suggested above, chant the mantras silently or use the note of G.

Planet ☿

Mercury is the planet of the Throat chakra.

Mercury is named after the fleet-footed messenger god who, like his Greek predecessor, Hermes, carried the healing caduceus staff with its entwined serpents (see page 98).

Mercury rules Gemini (22 May–21 June) and Virgo (24 August–22 September). Those born during this period generally find Throat chakra work easiest.

Throat chakra work is especially potent during those periods and on Wednesdays, which are ruled by Mercury. Mercury's caduceus induces sleep and so the planet like the god is an excellent focus for astral travel during sleep.

Beginning dreamwork

- Buy or make luminous planets to hang on your bedroom ceiling.

- Lie in the dark and focus on Mercury, visualising a doorway into the small, silvery planet.

- See yourself travelling through the night sky towards the planet, which grows larger and brighter until you are within not the physical plane, but the psychic one that exists at a higher vibration.

- If you look at your body, it may also glow silvery blue as you operate through this higher level of your body.

- Allow your mind to show you scenes until you fall asleep.

- As soon as you wake, whether or not you experienced a continuation of your Mercurian travel in sleep, re-create the scenario of astral travel, now moving through the early morning sky to Mercury.

- In time, you will enter an altered state of consciousness at night that will merge into the dream state and you will wake up in this semi-hypnotic state until you are ready to move into daytime consciousness.

- In time, you may wish to change the focus of Mercury for another scene but, while you are working with this chakra, the planet offers entry to a whole variety of astral dream states. You may even be aware of flying or floating, perhaps joined by a slender silver cord emanating from your Sacral chakra to your body.

Archangel

Raphael, angel of the Throat chakra, is the Archangel of the planet Mercury, the travellers' guide and the angel who offers healing to the planet and to humankind and all creatures on the face of the earth, in the skies and waters. He is also guardian of the young. Raphael is usually depicted with a pilgrim's stick, a wallet and a fish, showing the way and offering sustenance to all who ask. He is the angel of the night.

He heals technological and chemical pollution and the adverse effects of modern living.

You can focus your healing work on Raphael, calling him and being aware of blue light pouring from your own Throat chakra as you do so. You should also be aware of him answering.

You can use the focus of a blue candle or a deep blue beryl sphere and visualise Raphael in the light or the crystal, directing and amplifying the blue light that is manifest from your chakra. Whether you are healing yourself, a place, pollution in areas of natural beauty or someone else present or absent, the key is healing with the voice. The pure words will carry on the blue light the rays of energy necessary to heal body, mind and spirit and Raphael will speak through you, helping you to choose the right words.

Deities

Hathor, Thoth and other deities of truth and wisdom correspond to the Throat chakra.

There are many wise gods and goddesses associated with this chakra that is associated with truth, justice, right words and actions, but ancient Egypt is especially rich in them. My own favourite is Hathor, the ancient Egyptian goddess of truth, wisdom, joy, love, music, art and dance and protectress of women. She is said to bring husbands/wives to those who call on her and she is a powerful fertility goddess. Also worshipped as a sky goddess, Hathor is frequently shown wearing a sun disc held between the horns of a cow as a crown.

Her magic mirror reflects back all things in their true light. Her special symbols are gold, turquoise, roses, the colours red and orange and rose incense. Any of these can be used to endow you with her joyous but powerful presence, as can music and dance. In the modern world she is guardian of businesswomen. Fiercely protective in defence of her own, she is especially potent against physical and psychic attacks.

Thoth was the ancient Egyptian god of the Moon, wisdom and learning. He was also god of time, languages, law and mathematical calculations who invented the calendar and hieroglyphic writing. He is often depicted with the head of an ibis, though he was worshipped as a baboon in Hermopolis.

He was believed to be the father of healing wisdom, of magic and divination and his wisdom spread into the Western world through one of his descendants, the semi-legendary, first-century magician Hermes Trismegistos (Hermes was Thoth's Greek form who was called Mercury in Rome).

The following hieroglyphs, from ancient Egypt, are ones you can draw on stone or paint or etch on wood and use as a talisman to invoke clear and wise communication. Each hieroglyph was believed not only to represent but to contain the power it symbolises.

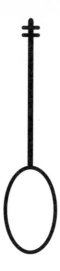

Nefer means happiness, good fortune and beauty, and is based on a musical instrument that resembled a primitive guitar. The perfect form and harmony of the instrument represented fulfilment and pleasure, and so is a sign of power associated with Hathor and the Throat chakra.

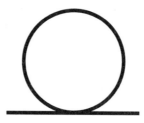

Shen represents the orbit of the Sun around the Earth and so was a symbol of time. As an amulet placed upon the dead, it promised eternal life so long as the Sun endured. And so again it is a symbol of power, related to Thoth who ruled time and also the Throat chakra that speaks of eternity once we rise beyond the limitations of linear time as we utilise higher chakra energies.

Creature

The creature associated with the Throat chakra is the elephant.

The elephant has great significance as a symbol of wisdom in both Western and Eastern mythology.

The Roman historian and chronicler Pliny believed that the elephant had religious feelings and worshipped the ancient deities of the Moon and stars. In Hinduism the elephant-headed Ganesha is god of wisdom and is always invoked at the beginning of any journey or before any important enterprise. Ganesha also rules learning and prosperity and is the remover of obstacles and deity of new beginnings.

The mighty trumpeting of the elephant also symbolises the power of this chakra. You can, therefore, roar out your own words of power alone in a clearing and, if you listen with your clairaudient or psychic ear, hear the returning affirmation of these powerful creatures hundreds or thousands of miles away.

Crystals

Throat chakra crystals are blue lace agate, blue beryl, lapis lazuli, blue quartz, sapphire and turquoise.

Each of these crystals can be placed in water for eight hours and the water will contain different properties related to this chakra according to the crystal used.

Blue lace agate heals sore throats, especially those caused by holding back what you need to say; they also soften harsh words and enable you to transform harshness or spite in the words of others.

Blue beryl enables you to speak prophetic words about global and personal issues and will suggest solutions.

Lapis lazuli, believed by the Sumerians and Babylonians to contain the souls of their gods, will enable you to tap into the wisdom of ancient times as you speak.

Blue quartz brings harmony in your words and defuses confrontation, also acting as a channel for wisdom from the higher chakras.

Sapphire aids clear communication and prevents guilt or sentiment creeping in from the lower chakras. It encourages nobility of words.

Turquoise as the power crystal helps when it is necessary to assume leadership and guide or teach others.

Incenses and oils

Fennel, ferns, lavender, lemongrass and valerian are related to the Throat chakra.

Each of these fragrances has its specific energies that form aspects of the chakras. Burn one or two separately and write, draw, paint or tell as a story on tape the feelings that each evokes. You may find that characters emerge that, on closer inspection, turn out to be aspects of yourself.

Herbs

Dill, lemon verbena, lily of the valley, parsley and peppermint are the herbs related to the Throat chakra.

Dry and chop any of these herbs; parsley and dill are probably the easiest to work with. Place about three tablespoons of the herbs into a ceramic dish; then sprinkle about half of the contents of the dish on to a stiff white sheet of paper over which you have painted a thin layer of paste.

Shake the paper, and then look, through half-closed eyes, at the picture that the herbs have created. Interpret the symbols as you would a story, and they will communicate hidden knowledge about a future path over which you had been puzzling.

Trees

Ash, hazel, poplar and sycamore are the trees corresponding to the Throat chakra.

Listen to the voices in the trees in different kinds of wind and in the rustling before rain. As you work with this chakra, you may hear with your inner or psychic ear snatches of poetry, short passages that you discover come from the Bible or the *I Ching*, the Chinese book of changes, songs and myths. You are now able to access the cosmic memory bank that tends to reveal knowledge in symbolic form.

Affirmation

The Throat chakra affirmation is 'I express'.

Working with the Throat chakra

Sacred geometry is the enclosure of a sacred space with geometric shapes and principles that have spiritual as well as mathematical significance. Though sacred geometry is used for secular purposes, its prime importance is in its spiritual symbolism, as a connection between the human and the divine.

A mandala is a geometric pattern that represents the sacred sphere, the union of the self and the universe. It features in the rituals and meditative practices in Hinduism, and many forms of Buddhism, especially Tibetan.

Mandalas are said to be the formal geometrical expression of sacred vibration or sacred sound and are created in many art forms as a way of expressing the path to the infinite. The mandala has also entered the Western mystical tradition, especially in more recent years, to express relationships between sacred symbols of, for example, the Kabbalah or alchemy.

During the 1930s Hans Jenny, a Swiss researcher, demonstrated that sound could not only cause matter to move, but create specific forms and shapes. Jenny also investigated sacred sounds. When he chanted Aum, 'om', the sound that is believed by Buddhists to bring the universe into being, into a device called a tonoscope, it produced first a circle, then created a mandala pattern.

Mandalas are primarily used for meditation either as an actual reproduction on a scroll or created in the mind by visualisation. They are also drawn in the earth or sand and are especially powerful in opening the Throat and the higher chakras. The earth or sand mandala is always completely destroyed after the ceremony.

A true mandala, which means circle in Sanskrit, has a perfect symmetrical form, concentrated around a central axis. From this central axis, the mandala is usually divided into four equal sections. Each of these divisions is itself made up of concentric circles and squares whose centres coincide with the centre of all the circles, thus creating an intricate design.

The mandala design is intended to guide an initiate into an altered state of awareness through contemplation, inwards to the sacred centre, the heart of silence.

There are incredibly complex mandalas that you can download from the Internet for personal use, but in practice even a child can draw a simple mandala.

On the next page is a simple design and a few suggestions of how to work. Again you can learn more of this art from Internet sites and books (see page 155).

Drawing and especially colouring a mandala is perhaps the best way to connect with sacred geometry and the inherent sacred sound in your mind. Remember those intricate patterns you coloured as a child and the incredible peace that came over you as you worked?

- Use white paper or card and colouring pens in rich, jewel colours.
- Draw around a dinner plate or use a compass to create an outer circle that fits comfortably within the page.

- Mark the centre of the circle and then draw a horizontal and a vertical line through the centre, to give four segments.
- Draw a single equal circle in each of the quadrants.
- In the centre of the original main circle draw a small circle and a large one that shares its central point. The larger circle should pass through the centre of the four small circles.

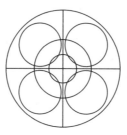

- Alternatively, create two concentric rings. Inside the second, draw a six-pointed star.
- Inside the star, draw another circle.

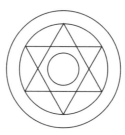

- If you remember to use a basic circle shape and divide it into four areas, keep your design symmetrical (each part is balanced) and use repetitive patterns to establish a rhythm that enables you to slip into a light trance state; you can create any form you wish.

EIGHT

The Brow Chakra or Ajna

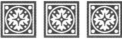

The Brow or Third Eye chakra is the gateway to light and control. As we climb ever higher up our cathedral tower, at last we reach the dome or square tower and we are flooded with light and impressions as the world is seen from high above. A few will want to venture right to the cross or the spire, but for many this is the peak of the journey. The psychic functions attributed to the Third Eye include clairvoyance and access to past lives. As integrator of the inner and outer world and other dimensions, it offers contact with angelic or spirit guides and the higher or evolved self.

Because this chakra is closer to the cosmos than the earth, inspiration comes increasingly filtered down through the Crown chakra and so there may be glimpses of divinity that, as yet, are not open to full control.

As this is the chakra of control, at this level you can make thoughts become reality through focusing your energies in ritual or visualisation, and many witches strive to attain this level of spiritual evolution in order to make spell-casting effective.

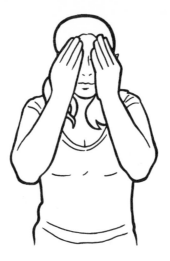

*Charging the
Brow chakra*

This does not mean, however, that witches are out there, casting evil spells. Even if you have worked on your spiritual development from when you were young, this chakra becomes most effective as you grow older and wiser. What is more, this chakra is at such a level of purity of intention that powers cannot be diverted into self-interest or wrong-doing, only healing and good works. You will also derive personal blessings through the threefold law whereby what you give out willingly returns with three times the power.

Sometimes this is regarded as the last human chakra before we merge with divine bliss, a state attained by spiritual masters and gurus or in death as our spirits leave as they first came, through the Crown chakra. However, others, myself included, believe that it is because we can at least partially work through the Crown chakra that we are able to understand a little of divinity and tap into our own divine core, the god or goddess within, during this lifetime (see page 110).

The Brow chakra is the channel for wisdom, past, present and future. The cosmic memory bank we first utilised in the Throat chakra now becomes far more accessible and, though we may still work with divinatory forms such as the Tarot, the cards act as a focus for clairvoyance that extends far beyond their accepted meanings.

Clairvoyance, or clear-seeing with the psychic or Third Eye, bears no relation to physical acuity, as many blind people are very clairvoyant.

It is said that clairvoyant abilities reside in the Third Eye. This is biologically associated with the pineal gland located in the back of the brain almost in the centre of the head, that is believed to have shrunk during human evolution. Early humans were hypothesised to have breathed through this gland rather than the nose and mouth. This gland thus operated as a constant doorway to the world and was said to connect people to the energies around rather than isolating them within their skulls. The Third Eye is also a name given to the Brow chakra, a psychic energy centre that is linked with all forms of spiritual and psychic functioning.

Whereas the Throat chakra is biased towards words, with this chakra it is images that are the most important. You will find that as this chakra is activated any form of scrying (picturing images within a reflective surface) becomes increasingly accurate and draws on the universal images of myth and legend we last spontaneously used in childhood.

Location of the Brow chakra

The Brow chakra is situated just above the bridge of the nose in the centre of the brow. It controls the eyes, ears and both hemispheres of the brain, and radiates into the central cavity of the brain.

It is here that the *ida* and *pingala*, the left lunar and right solar channels that began in the Root chakra and spiralled their way up the chakra system like the caduceus of Hermes, finally merge with the *sushumna* central column. Blockages here can result in blurred vision without reason, headaches and migraines, and blocked sinuses as well as earache. On a psychological level, insomnia or nightmares can result from blockages.

Brow chakra correspondences

Colour

Indigo is the colour that corresponds to the Brow chakra.

Use coloured Perspex, indigo candles or a shaded light bulb to filter indigo light upon you before you sleep to filter out the sensations that have flooded your mind through your eyes and ears throughout the day. This allows the psychic sensations residing in the Brow or Third Eye chakra to lead you gently into the night and peaceful dreams, clearing away any blockages or pollution while you sleep.

Element

The element corresponding to the Brow chakra is light.

Creating a light body

This method is especially good for opening and clearing the Third Eye but has a beneficial effect on all the chakras from Root to Crown.

- Sit in sunlight, or any natural light, however dull the day. Some practitioners work in darkness or by candlelight, but I believe that natural light is the transmitter of spiritual light.

- Sit so that your feet are touching the floor, either in a chair or on the floor, with your palms facing upwards.

- Visualise white light pouring into your body through your auric field from all around, but focus on your feet, and feel as well as see the light rising from the soles of your feet like warm liquid, pure gold from the Earth.

- Focus next on your ankles and allow them to fill with light. Be aware of the gentle pressure as the light moves upwards through your ankles and to the perineum so that your Root chakra is not red but golden.

- Next move your attention to the Crown of your head and be aware of pure white light entering through the fontanelle and spreading through the skull down through the ears and eyes.

- Turn next to the light ascending slowly from below and the continuing rising of the light that gets ever paler as the white light comes downwards.

- Each time light from below or above reaches a chakra, you will experience a lovely warm swirling and the streams moving closer, extending out to your arms and hands via the Heart chakra.

- Once the light gains impetus, relax and enjoy the sensations as the light entering each chakra simultaneously adds to the upward and downward flow, ending as a glorious waterfall somewhere between the Throat and Heart chakras.

- Sit quietly and let the light flow within you and around you.

You can carry out this ritual daily or whenever you feel depleted and out of touch with your psyche.

The energies will disperse naturally throughout your physical body and the layers of the Etheric body. If you look in the mirror you will see with your inner or even physical eye not only a luminous aura, but a circle of light around your Third Eye.

Symbol

Entwined snakes on a caduceus are the symbol of the Brow chakra.

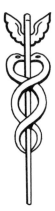

The symbol may also incorporate eagle wings signifying wisdom or a circle representing the void, with a lotus petal either side to represent the synthesis of male and female, positive and negative (see page 81).

Mantra sound

Aum (pronounced Om) is the mantra sound related to the Brow chakra.

According to Buddhist belief, this is the sound that brought the universe into being. This is a very special mantra and will resound through all the lower chakras and so can be used to revitalise them all.

Planet ♃

Jupiter, known as the sky-Father, is the planet related to the Brow chakra.

As the supreme Roman god and ruler of the universe, Jupiter was a role model for the ideal emperor who was both general, statesman and spiritual leader (the reality invariably fell rather short).

Like his Greek counterpart Zeus, Jupiter controlled the thunderbolts, which were carried by his eagle, the king and noblest of the birds. However, he ruled not despotically, but as the chief of a triumvirate of gods, the others of whom were Juno, his consort, and Minerva, goddess of wisdom, who made up the feminine principle of deeper, more instinctual wisdom.

Jupiter rules Sagittarius (23 November–21 December) and is co-ruler of Pisces (19 February–20 March) which are good times for Brow chakra work as is Thursday, his special day. Those born at these times will generally find it easiest to work with Brow chakra energies.

The planet is perhaps more inspirational than the god, who could be cruel and domineering. It represents an increase in abundance and prosperity, idealism and the expansion of horizons. It is this aspect that is related to the Brow chakra.

If possible, climb mountains or high hills or tall buildings with sacred connections, temples, cathedrals or monuments. This time look not downwards but upwards, and allow your mind to merge with the sky.

Make pictures in the clouds as the Druids did and use the images not to answer immediate personal questions but to see clearly the paths ahead, not only for yourself but also for the world. You may be rewarded by a quick glimpse of a future time, perhaps of yourself reborn or a descendant who carried your genes or of wider vistas. Record these in your chakra journal.

Archangel

Sachiel, angel of the Brow chakra, is the Archangel of the planet Jupiter, the divine benefactor. He is the angel of charity who says that only by giving freely to others will our own needs be met. He works constantly to help others and to improve the lives of humankind. He restores run-down areas or cities where employment has been lost, blending new skills with traditional knowledge.

His special role is to help you to move closer to your own personal guardian angel or spirit guide.

Finding your angel

It has been said that our personal angels are the essence of what we are at our most evolved, our higher selves. Others believe that angels are separate entities that have never lived on Earth, but are of a higher order. Some of these angels choose to guide a particular person or act as guardians to a city or even a nation. It is said that we all have a guardian angel. As your Brow chakra is activated, so this contact will become easier and through your angel you can channel messages from an even more evolved being of light.

- Just before you go to bed on a Thursday, light an indigo candle and look into the flame.
- Let your eyes half-close and see the aura of the candle expanding to fill the darkness.
- Ask Sachiel if it is right for you to see your personal guide.

- Close your eyes, open them, look into the flame, blink and you may see him or her either in your mind's vision or in the candle aura. You may also see the shadowy image of Sachiel behind.

- Angels can take many forms and yours will take that which is right for you, whether a golden angel with wings or a wise man or woman in a brown robe.

- Touch your Third Eye and then your Heart chakra with your right hand. The angel will touch his or hers with the left, completing the union and establishing the sign you can make unobtrusively when you feel the need for your angel to move close and offer wisdom or protection.

- Leave the candle to burn down in a safe place and thank Sachiel for his help, promising to plant some seeds on waste land or clear litter the next day to help Sachiel in his work.

If you carry out this ritual regularly, you will find that you see your special angel in more detail. You may also hear a soft but clear voice in your ear that is your own and yet richer, calmer and one you have heard a thousand times in your dreams or on the wind.

Deities

Nut, Shiva/Shakti and Horus are the deities of the Brow chakra.

Nut, the ancient Egyptian sky goddess, was called the mother of the gods and of all living things. She was invoked in life and death by humans for protection. Nut's body, covered in stars, was arched over the Earth, protecting it, as she touched it with her fingertips and toes, and lay over her husband Seb the Earth god.

She was the mother of Ra, the Sun god, and early myths tell how he returned to her womb every night to be reborn at dawn.

Shiva/Shakti, the male and female central deities in Hinduism are united in a single figure known as Sakti Hakini or Ardhanarishvara, with the male part of the figure on the right and the female on the left. Their energies are permanently fused and synthesised, for this chakra marks the end of duality.

Horus was the ancient Egyptian sky god, represented as a falcon or a falcon-headed man. His eyes were the Sun and Moon and his wings could extend across the entire heavens.

One of the most famous symbols is the hieroglyph of the eye of Horus, which is associated with the Third Eye or Brow chakra.

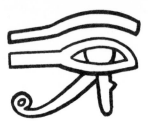

The hieroglyph represents the white or Sun (Ra) eye, and marks the full power of the Sun. Therefore it is empowering as well as protective, and guards against deception since it is the eye of truth.

Opening the Third Eye

- Draw an eye of Horus in the centre of your Brow with an indigo lipstick or eye shadow.

- Light indigo candles in a circle around you and, closing your eyes, focus on the light through the Third Eye centre. In your mind, picture the radiance from the candles entering through the eye of Horus as you inhale and exhale steadily.

- Allow images to form in your mind. These may be single symbols, faces of people or entire figures, usually with a distinctive unusual item of clothing or feature that, because they are moving in the vision, is prominent. You probably will not know the faces.

- Do not try to attach words to the visions rather, as when you were a child, allow the imaging part of your brain that is connected with higher and deeper wisdom to take control.

- When you are ready, open your physical eyes and using paints or colouring pens reproduce the symbols or figures that you saw. You will find that your artistic abilities are greater than usual, even if this is not a particular talent. Do not worry about the skill, however; rather record faithfully what you saw with your clairvoyant eye.

Most psychic artists have highly evolved Third Eyes and draw people from other dimensions who may be deceased relations of friends or even strangers who are yet to cross their path.

You may see guides or guardian spirits and this is a way that your own guides may contact you. If so, you will have a sense of recognition.

Carry out this exercise once a week, or when you feel the urge, and you will find that the symbols, however unusual, occur in your life within a few days. If you see strange people, you may find that a colleague or friend mentions that he or she has a relation with those odd attributes.

In time you will not need to draw the eye or even to set aside a special time. Your clairvoyance not only of other dimensions but of facts about people you meet for the first time will become increasingly accurate as this psychic centre evolves.

Creature

The cobra corresponds to the Brow chakra.

In the Root chakra, we met the serpent and the snake goddesses. Here, at the higher level, it is the cobra, most magnificent of snakes, that rears high to strike and remains sacred in a number of cultures including those of Egypt and India.

The cobra was associated with the Egyptian goddess Uadjet, pictured as a winged and crowned cobra, a goddess of the Underworld, justice and truth.

She was both protector and destroyer, spitting poison at any who would do the pharaoh harm, or burning them with her eyes of fire. She also administered the death sting when the pharaoh's appointed time on Earth was over. She guided souls through the Underworld, showing them how to avoid the snares of the spirit serpents.

Her name means the fiery eye of Ra, the Sun god with whom she was associated.

You can work with the symbol of the healing caduceus of the Egyptian Thoth, the double entwined snake of the classical Hermes and Mercury's caduceus, often a living, growing staff.

The snake forms two circles, the interlinked cycles of good and evil, life and death, light and darkness. The wings on the caduceus are for wisdom. Use this as an amulet etched in indigo wax (see page 56) or painted on a crystal. Alternatively, make yourself a caduceus staff from wood or metal and place it at your door so that only the higher energies will enter.

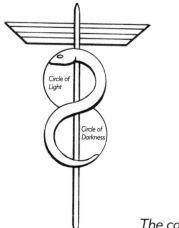

The caduceus of Hermes

Crystals

Amethyst, azurite, kunzite, lapis lazuli, sodalite and sugilite relate to the Brow chakra.

Sharpen your mind, psychic awareness and intuition, and improve your memory by rubbing a vibrant Brow crystal, such as a deep amethyst or opaque sugilite, clockwise directly on to your Brow in the place of the Third Eye and let the sensations come. You may see soft rainbow colours or hear faint sounds, even music. You may momentarily connect with both past and future.

Incenses and oils

Copal, mistletoe, sage, sandalwood, sweetgrass and thyme are associated with the Brow chakra.

- Light any of these as incense sticks and circle anti-clockwise over your Brow chakra three times to remove the blockages caused by daily life.

- Then sit quietly in the fragrance and allow images to form.

- You may discover that some images appear regularly to you. This indicates that they have special significance in your immediate future.

- Keep an alphabetical list of these recurring images in your journal, together with what they mean to you.

- If you look at conventional symbol interpretation books, you will be surprised at how similar your meanings are. As you work with this chakra so do you spontaneously tap ever more easily into the collective wisdom of humankind that is the source for mythology throughout the world.

Exploring past worlds

- Light one of your Brow chakra incenses or oils, and place safely so you cannot burn yourself if you drift into sleep.

- Lie where you are comfortable and rest a dark amethyst or sodalite on your Brow chakra.

- Close your eyes and softly begin to count backwards from thirty to nought.

- As you count, visualise walking down steps and along a path until you come to a wood.

- By now you will have finished counting so begin to describe the scene aloud – the creatures you see, the people you meet and any buildings you enter.

- You will meet a guide who is someone you recognise from dreams, perhaps the wise figure you drew when you were working with the eye of Horus or were shown by Sachiel. This guardian will keep you safe and show you the way back when you decide to leave the world you are entering.

- It can be helpful to set a tape running so that you can recall the details or ask a friend to work with you and guide you through the exercise.

- You will identify someone who resembles you or with whom you feel affinity.

- Watch and follow. These characters belong to a past time and cannot see you, but if you watch and listen, you may begin to understand things about your present life and relationships.

- Whatever happens, nothing can hurt you. If you begin to feel uneasy or that it is time to go, your guide will take you back to the edge of the wood where you can begin counting, this time from one to thirty. When you reach thirty, you will find yourself lying on the bed. Before you depart, the guide may have a special message for you or may remain silent.

- When you are ready, open your eyes and remove the crystal from your Brow. Place it beneath your pillow.

- Whether what you saw was an actual past world or symbolic, allow impressions to come and go. You may continue the journey in your dreams.

Do not carry out this exercise more than once a month. You may visit other times in the same life or different periods, but your guide will always be there.

Herbs

Agrimony, borage, cinquefoil, coltsfoot and hyssop are the herbs of the Brow chakra.

Grow any of these herbs in pots and, when you feel lacking in inspiration, place one of the pots in your work space or in the area where you work at home. Alternatively, keep a ceramic bowl of the dried herbs to rub on your forehead when you feel confused by conflicting advice or sensations. Avoid doing this in pregnancy or if you have any chronic medical conditions.

Trees

Beech, cedar and oak are the trees that relate to the Brow chakra.

The trees of the Brow chakra can aid you in manifesting thought forms. The space between two oak trees, in particular, is said to be the gateway to other dimensions.

Working with thought forms

- Find a space between two trees, whether oaks or another ancient species.
- Moving in a clockwise direction, scatter a circle of Brow chakra herbs within this space, beginning in the north. Then sit in the south facing north, the direction of magical insights.
- Hold between your hands a symbol of what it is you want to bring from the thought plane to actuality, preferably something that will bring happiness to other people as well as yourself.
- Then begin to move around the circle, chanting and dancing, still holding the symbol, saying:

    Tree power at this hour,

    Bring to me what I see.

- Move and chant faster until you feel you can contain the power no more. Leap into the air thrusting the symbol high and then swoop to the ground still holding it.
- Bury the symbol at or close to the spot where you have been working and then move anti-clockwise around the circle saying:

    May the circle be uncast but not broken,

    Blessings be.

When you go home, begin practical steps to help the thought form manifest more easily. This may involve writing letters or making phone calls concerning your wish. You may make applications or work on money-spinning schemes, searching the Internet for relevant information. The more active you are, the more substance the thought form will have to which to attach itself.

Affirmation

'I see clearly' is the affirmation associated with the Brow chakra.

Working with the Brow chakra

One of the best ways of developing the Brow chakra is by creating an indigo pyramid and sitting or meditating within it. Purple pyramids have been used for developing psychic powers and for healing for years, but came to the attention of the UK media when the Duchess of York used one when she visited a clairvoyant/ healer.

Experiments demonstrate that sitting under a pyramid measurably increases the amplitude and frequency of *Alpha* and *Theta* brain waves that are naturally present in states of meditation and altered consciousness. This occurs even when subjects are blindfolded and unaware that an open pyramid structure has been lowered over them. Alpha brain waves help efficient functioning of the Third Eye.

An indigo pyramid seems to enhance these powers even further by clearing and strengthening the Brow or Third Eye chakra through which psychic functions operate.

The Great Pyramid of Cheops at Giza in Egypt, constructed circa 2700 BC by Pharaoh Khufu (Cheops in Greek) is the most magical of all pyramids.

Sitting inside a scale model of the Great Pyramid that is draped with purple or holding a miniature pyramid in amethyst and gazing into it, improves telepathic communication, clairaudience, clairvoyance and mediumship.

Sleeping with a small pyramid beneath the bed not only increases energy levels the next day in many people, but brings predictive dreams and out-of-body sensations, especially ones connected with past lives.

Pyramids also accelerate self-healing and natural growth in people, plants and animals.

Making a pyramid

- Providing a model pyramid is constructed as nearly as possible to a scale based on the Cheops pyramid, a home-made pyramid can be constructed of almost any material and any size, from a pyramid large enough to sit in or lie under to one small enough to hold in the hand.

- The Great Pyramid itself has four sides, each measuring 230 metres (755 feet) at the base, and is 147 metres (481 feet) high at the summit. A scale model using these proportions can be created, using a calculator. For example, a representative tepee 1.47 metres high, with sides 2.3 metres at the base could be created.

- You can drape it with indigo cloth or stick indigo-painted paper to the basic frame.

- The frame can be as simple as an adapted clothes dryer or a huge cardboard box, painted or coloured in indigo.

- Purple Perspex pyramids or pyramid frames can also be obtained easily and relatively cheaply through New Age stores by mail order and via the Internet.

- It is a tool that you can use for many forms of psychic work, and using one even for a few minutes will offer almost instant cleansing and empowerment to the Brow chakra.

- If, however, you want an instant pyramid, other pyramid shapes can also heighten psychic powers. You could drape an indigo blanket over a child's toy tepee, or pin indigo material from the bedroom ceiling in a pyramid shape and attach it to the bed frame.

- Alternatively, because your spiritual powers are evolving, you could visualise yourself inside a purple crystalline pyramid of the kind reputed to exist in Atlantis, or picture the actual Cheops pyramid, dyed purple with the setting sun.

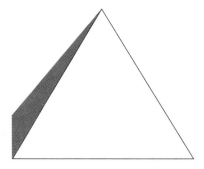

The model pyramid. Prepare four sides and stick them together to produce the pyramid as shown (the shaded area shows how the flap has been folded under one side)

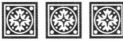

NINE

The Crown Chakra
or Sahasrara

This is the chakra of union and bliss.

White, the source of pure light (all the other colours combined), pours upwards and outwards into the cosmos, and downwards and inwards from the cosmos back into the Crown. It represents wisdom, a deep and all-embracing wisdom.

Sahasrara means one thousand, and refers to the number of petals on the symbolic lotus chakra that whirls so fast that there is no beginning and no end. When energy flows freely, although we still follow our everyday life, that life is touched with grace and beauty and an awareness that we are not only connected to all Nature and existence, as we discovered in the Heart chakra, but that every part of that creation contains a spark of divinity and so is sacred.

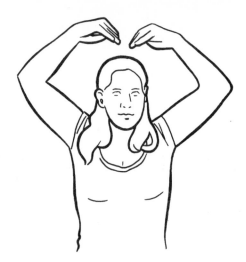

*Charging the
Crown chakra*

When we finally reach the most slender part of our cathedral, the cross or the top of the tower, we are still connected to earth but are closer to the heavens. Many of our basic fears – of our own mortality and of being alone – fade and lose their thrall. When we die, our spirit returns to the source of divinity through the Crown to merge with cosmic bliss or to return to learn more lessons, if you believe in karma and reincarnation. Alternatively, it may rise to a place of joy and peace with the source of divinity where the essential self and personality lives on in the form of the Etheric or Spirit body. The Crown chakra relates to the highest layer of this body (see page 22) and some people believe that it is this part alone that survives death. The truth is that we do not know.

However, from my own research and the studies of others into near-death experiences, death-bed visions and those who see a deceased relation return in spirit form, I am convinced that some or all of the Etheric body does survive death.

Visions of hell belong to the guilt and prohibitions of theologians who operate only through their lower chakras. I believe that for those who are truly wicked, their spirits do ascend into the light, but they are so surrounded by their own darkness, they cannot see it and so wander forever – or until they are enlightened and can make atonement.

In the Crown chakra, the Kundalini energy from the Root chakra merges with the Shiva or cosmic energy, and Earth and sky become one; all the other chakra energies are integrated and polarities and conflicting energies merge.

As a result of working with this chakra, harmony and highest healing energies will pass down through your other chakras and permeate every aspect of your being and your life. You may find that you have glimpses or momentary awareness of your connection with the whole universe through mystical or what psychologists call peak experiences. This chakra is primarily about merging, about *being* rather than *doing* and this is reflected in the activities connected with it.

Location of the Crown chakra

The Crown chakra is situated at the top of the head in the centre where the three main bones of the skull fuse at the anterior fontanelle. It extends beyond the Crown and some locate the centre about three finger-breadths above the top of the head. It rules the brain, body and psyche. It connects the highest or most evolved part of the self, wherein resides our personal core of divinity – that ultimately connects to the source of divinity itself.

Blockages here can result in headaches and migraines, in inefficient functioning of the immune system and a tendency to forgetfulness and minor accidents. On a psychological level, blockages are manifest as a sense of alienation from the world.

Crown chakra correspondences

Colour

Violet merging into white/gold is the colour associated with the Crown chakra.

Bright sunlight can allow us to experience the brilliant white colour of the Crown chakra.

Ascending the steps of light

- Find a flight of steps, perhaps in the grounds of an old house or cathedral, the steep part of an old town or a botanical garden. My own favourite spot is the steep white steps up to the Cathedral of Sacre Coeur in Paris, itself built on top of a high hill. From the steps themselves you get a vista of the whole city, and because of the design of the building you can walk up a number of steps before entering the shade.

- Work in sunlight and walk towards the increasing light, so that there is a shimmering haze.

- As you ascend, blend into the sunlight so that your body is shimmering inside and say nothing, focus on nothing – just experience the warmth and brilliance.

- Afterwards, sit at the top of the steps and you may, in the haze in front of your eyes, be rewarded with a momentary vision of a light being or experience a sense of being one with the light.

Element

Spirit or ether is associated with the Crown chakra.

Spirit is created by the synthesis of the four elements and the integration of all aspects of existence into a greater and higher state, described sometimes as the still point of the turning world, or the silence between two waves.

If we sit in deep countryside at night with only the calling of the night birds, on a lonely shore as the sea rises and falls, in a shadowy deserted rural church or in a city centre on a quiet, early morning, the stillness can fill us with a deep peace that is almost unearthly. It not only carries us beyond time, but dissolves our own separate self. Such moments are rare, but it is possible to induce this state that allows energies to flow more easily through the Crown chakra from above and below, allowing us to merge with the collective energies of the universe and lose our sense of aloneness and alienation.

Stilling the mind

You may wish to begin by grounding (see page 64) and centring yourself (see page 75).

- Then still your body by finding a place, preferably in sunlight, but if not, anywhere you are warm and comfortable where you can sit undisturbed.

- Do nothing. This can be incredibly hard for many of us, myself included, as there are a thousand and one lists to write, phone calls to make, unfinished chores to do and books to read. But just for a while, be still. Do not even listen to music.

- Try this for five or ten minutes and gradually the racing thoughts will also still. Take off your watch so you do not time yourself or worry about where you should be next.

- The next stage is to still the mind and gently push away the racing thoughts, the mental shopping lists, the rehearsed conversations – in my case the chapter I am writing in my head if I am not careful, even when I am supposed to be meditating.
- Let each thought come and gently push it away as though launching a toy boat on a pond. Watch as it sails away.

The most successful instant method I have encountered is one that I have already described in this book. Picture a sky full of stars and watch them one by one going out until you are enclosed in a velvety blackness. Or visualise a jug of clear water you are pouring into a stream drop by drop until it is gone and there is only the rhythm of the water. Another method is to visualise sitting on an empty train that slows down and suddenly stops in the middle of the countryside and gradually all sound and motion ceases. Alternatively (if you enjoy flying), imagine yourself in the state of being alone in a half-empty plane with sunlight filtering through the windows, flying though cotton wool clouds as the strain of getting to the airport recedes and the arrival is hours away.

The last two are especially good if you really are on that empty train or plane. I attained the latter state after I had been caught in the Los Angeles earthquake in 1994 and after a diversion found myself with a whole bank of seats to myself on a long flight from Seattle to Heathrow. Having had no sleep for 24 hours but having been through such a traumatic experience when the floor beneath my hotel room shook, I became part of the plane interior and between sleeping and waking lost all sense of self until we landed ten hours later. It was a surreal but quite magical experience.

Symbol

The circle is the symbol of the Crown chakra.

The circle sometimes contains a single black dot to indicate the First Principle, the source of existence. The circle represents spirit and the whole cosmos, everything that is. The dot is the seed of new life, the limitless given form.

Mantra sound

Silence corresponds to the Crown chakra.

This is the Zen Buddhist concept of clapping with one hand or striking a note, perhaps the B note that corresponds to the violet Crown chakra vibration, and allowing the sound to fade into silence. It is beyond even reciting in your mind a mantra, though you might wish to make aloud a single 'Aum', the sound that brought the universe into being, gradually trailing into silence.

Planet ☉

The Sun is the planet related to the Crown chakra.

The glyph of the Sun corresponds exactly with the symbol of the Crown chakra.

The Sun rules Leo (23 July–23 August) and those born at this time will generally find it easiest to work with Crown chakra energies. Others will tune into the energies on Sundays and during Leo.

Making Sun water

Sun water is most potent when made on the morning of the longest day, the Summer Solstice, around June 21 (21 December in the Southern hemisphere), during a partial eclipse or, if you are lucky enough to have one in your region, a total eclipse of the Sun. However, you can also make Sun water any day from dawn till noon.

- Fill a brass or gold-coloured bowl or one of clear crystal (the kind used as old-fashioned fruit bowls) with pure spring water (you can use bottled still mineral water, many of which come from former sacred springs). Otherwise use rainwater collected in a vessel placed on a low roof or a water butt.

- Add three clear crystal quartz and, if you wish, surround the bowl with sunshine yellow flowers.

- Leave from dawn until noon or when the Sun is directly overhead in your time zone. (You can put the bowl out overnight if you do not wish to get up early. Cover it with fine mesh to keep out any pollution.)

- Bottle the water in tiny clear glass or gold-coloured bottles with stoppers. You can keep a few in the fridge to drink.

- Add a few drops of your Sun water into baths, splash on your brow and hairline if you feel stressed or spaced out and sip before working with the Crown chakra. You can sprinkle a few drops on any Sun herbs that are wilting.

Archangel

St Michael, angel of the Crown chakra, is the Archangel of the Sun, of light and the warrior angel. As commander of the heavenly hosts, Michael, usually pictured with a sword, drove Satan and his fallen angels out of the celestial realms.

You can feel his presence most vividly on a May morning, famed for the St Michael sunrise when, all along a ley line in England from St Michael's Mount in Cornwall to East Anglia, the Sun can be seen rising over the Sun churches named after St Michael and St George (formerly linked with the Northern Sun god Og), like beacons.

- Whether or not you are a Christian, go to one of his special places: St Michael's Mount in Cornwall or Mont St Michel, the fairy-tale castle island on the borders of Brittany and Normandy. This has a church on top and a golden statue of Michael with his flaming sword pointing along the ancient ley that runs from Mount Carmel in Israel to St Michael's Mount and thereon along the St Michael line, passing through the megalithic Avebury.

- Visit one of his cathedrals or mighty churches, usually built on the site of a temple to a Sun god or goddess or often close to an ancient indigenous Sun site in the New World.

- Stand on top of a hill or in a desert place or plain and see the hugeness of the Sun and Michael in the flaming sunrise, at noon trailing light beams and, at sunset, magnificent in scarlet and purple.

St Michael is the most powerful of all the Archangels and you will probably be aware of his presence only momentarily, in one of those moments in and out of time, described by T.S. Eliot as 'sudden in a shaft of sunlight' and 'costing not less than everything'. For as your Crown chakra floods with celestial light, whatever you call this divine power, at this moment you surrender your will to the power of the light and afterwards you cannot remain unchanged.

Deities

God, the Goddess and Divine Light are associated with the Crown chakra.

Connecting with the divinity within

Within us all is the spark of divinity. Whether we believe in a supreme God or All-Father or the Goddess as the Monad, the one undifferentiated source of light and life, or a power that cannot be called by any name or be known, let alone described in terms of a god or goddess, we carry within us the seed of that divinity.

It is that core that comes with us when we are incarnated and remains our essential self whether through one or many lifetimes.

But this sense of being divine can become buried in the modern frantic world and with it the sense of responsibility we have as caretakers of the earth with a duty to respect the divinity of every other species in existence.

Opening this chakra makes that connection and conversely making the connection activates the chakra. The Native North American people acknowledge we are only one part of the sacred web and this concept we worked with in the Heart chakra. Now, however, it is the sanctity of each species including our own, the god/dess within that is of importance.

The Australian Aborigines believe that we are descended from plants as well as from animals and birds and anthropology is increasingly discovering the wisdom of these ancient peoples.

You can if you wish carry these stages out at separate times or devote a morning or afternoon to greeting your fellow creatures one after the other. It is a good method if you are feeling out of touch with yourself and with the world.

- Begin with the Stone people. Find a stone on a riverbank, on a seashore, on a hillside or in an urban square. They are all precious.

- Lift your stone to what natural light there is and say:

  You are divine, you are my brother and sister,

  so am I divine and welcome you in our mutual sanctity.

  I offer you my protection and ask yours.

- Touch your Heart, your Throat, your Brow and finally your hairline for the Crown chakra with the stone as you speak.

- Return it to where you found it.

- Move next to the Plant people and find a tall plant or flower, making sure the one you choose is not an irritant or poison.

- Take a single petal or leaf and again touch your Heart, Throat, Brow and Crown chakras, saying as before:

  You are divine, you are my brother and sister,

  so am I divine and welcome you in our mutual sanctity.

  I offer you my protection and ask yours.

- Return the leaf or petal to the earth next to the plant.

- Next find the Tree people and, leaning against the trunk of a tree, touch it and then in turn your Heart, Throat etc, repeating the words. Alternatively, you can use a small frond you find lying near the tree or pick a small leafy twig, again returning it to the ground.

- Next find an insect or a butterfly settled on a plant and this time touch the creature's aura, not it, before it flies or crawls away (you may find the insect or butterfly remains motionless) and touch the upper four chakras with the auric essence, speaking as before.

- For the Winged and Four-legged people you can use a pet or visit an animal or bird sanctuary where there are tame creatures, but you may prefer to work with the essence of the aura, without touching the animal.

- For fish, visit an aquarium where certain fish such as koi or rays are amenable to being touched during feeding, and repeat the ritual.

- When you have finished, you may wish to do something practical to help one of your fellow species under threat.

Creature

The ouroboros is the creature related to the Crown chakra.

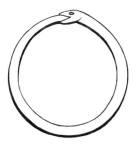

We have met the serpent in the Root and the Brow chakras because it is so fundamental to chakra work. Here, however, is the most magical of serpents, found in the legends of many lands curled around the world.

Mediaeval alchemists portrayed the ouroboros, the snake swallowing its own tail, a symbol of endless cycles of time, birth and rebirth unbroken. Because of the shape, it promises long life and protects against all destructive, divisive forces.

You can make an amulet by weaving or plaiting dried grasses, perhaps bound around a thin gold bracelet or ring, metal of the Sun and this chakra.

Crystals

White and purple banded amethyst, diamond, pearl, crystal quartz and brilliant purple sugilite are associated with the Crown chakra.

Merging with the crystal

This is a method I use both for teaching crystal healing and divination, but it is also a valuable way of softening the separate boundaries of the self and merging with cosmic energies. (See page 156 for details of my books in which I use this technique for healing and divination.) If you use a large piece of unpolished quartz or amethyst, you can gaze into it afterwards and momentarily intuit the world from a different perspective.

- Wait until after dusk and surround your crystal with a horseshoe of purple candles and burn frankincense or another Crown chakra incense stick or cone to enhance your psychic awareness. Myrrh and sandalwood are also very potent.

- Gaze into the crystal and very slowly breathe in the coloured light through your nose and gently exhale any darkness or greyness through your mouth as a sigh.

- As you continue to breathe in the crystalline light, draw it around you and visualise yourself within a huge crystal through which the purple candlelight filters.

- Imagine your boundaries dissolving so that the crystalline radiance can flow freely within as well as around you.

- Hear the crystal breathing and feel on a psychic level the gentle vibration it makes as though it was your own heartbeat.

- Allow images to form of the deep volcanic fires, the rushing waters, the cool breezes and the rich soil that caused its formation and of the land from which the crystal came.

- Now let the images fade and, as you continue to breathe gently and regularly, be filled with the light and the sound and the rootedness of the crystal in the Earth, with the Sky, the Fire and the Water.

- Feel its energies melting any rigidity remaining within you and filling you with a clear liquid energy that gently swirls and spirals.

- When you are ready, gently draw your boundaries around you again so that the crystalline light forms a halo around you and then separates so you are holding the crystal and can still feel its energies.

Incenses and oils

Benzoin, frankincense, gum Arabic (acacia), desert and mountain sage (sage brush), neroli and orange are associated with the Crown chakra.

Smudging

The following ritual involves smudging the seven directions to contact the still centre. Smudging can also be used to purify the chakras (see page 137).

This ritual is best done with a sage brush smudge stick, which can be bought from general New Age and even health stores as well as Native American suppliers. Rosemary and juniper fronds, tied tightly together with non-flammable twine at regular intervals along the stick and dried, also make excellent smudge sticks. The seven directions – east, west, north, south, down, up and the self as centre – symbolise the seven chakras and you can think of each one as you work. Smudging works beautifully in the open air if you are not in a windy place. If the smudge stick goes out, simply relight it, saying:

Blessings be, joined are we

and continue. The smoke will ascend on the sunlight. However, you can equally well work indoors, preferably not near soft furnishings or on carpet. (See page 156 for details of books on smudging, as this is such a valuable technique in chakra work.)

- Light the tip of your smudge stick and, when the flame dies down, blow on it gently until the end glows.
- Visualise a circle around yourself and face the east.
- Hold the smudge stick horizontally directly in front of you and smudge a small circle in the air, saying:

I join myself with the powers of the east, enter and empower,

I ask you, spirit guardians.

- Face south, west and north in turn, smudging a clockwise circle in each position and repeating the chant for the guardians of each direction.
- Then crouch down and point the smudge to the ground (down), smudging another clockwise circle, this time around your feet, saying:

I join myself with the powers of the Earth, enter and empower,

I ask you, Guardian and Mother.

- Hold your smudge stick at waist level and smudge around yourself (the centre), saying:

    I am part of the great chain of life. Let all flow

    within me as I flow with it.

- Finally raise your smudge high, and then lower it slightly, drawing a clockwise circle of smoke, two or three finger-breadths above your head, the centre of the Crown chakra, saying:

    I join myself with the powers of the Sky, enter and empower,

    I ask you, Guardian and Father.

- Smudge two more clockwise circles over the Crown and let your smudge burn through on a ceramic dish or in a container.

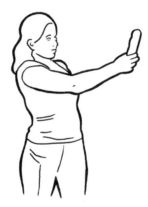

Herbs

Bay, chamomile, juniper, marigold, rosemary and St John's wort are the herbs of the Crown chakra.

Creating a Sun circle herb garden

You can create a special herb patch even in a small garden in the shape of the Sun/Crown chakra glyph by planting a circle of Sun/Crown chakra herbs or any other small sunshine yellow or orange flowers. In the centre, place a tiny crystal quartz to form the dot. If you do not have a garden, you can use an indoor tub or individual pots in a circle with Crown chakra crystals in the middle.

Trees

Banana, bay, chestnut/horse chestnut, laurel and orange are the trees that relate to the Crown chakra.

In earlier times it was believed that the world tree formed the axis of the world. In societies where traditions have continued unbroken for thousands of years, shamans or the magical priest/healers of a community still ascend the world tree in a trance to visit the upper realms. Here they seek healing and counsel for the people from the wise spirits and ancestors and ask the Mistress of the Animals to send the herds for hunting.

- When the Sun is overhead at noon (GMT), look up through one of the Sun trees or a tall, large, well-foliaged tree and feel the power of the Sun filtering through the leaves.

- Do not look directly at the Sun.

- Holding the trunk, close your eyes and in your mind's eye, climb up the tree towards the Sun and move through the brilliance into the Upper Realms.

- Through the brilliance you may see beings of pure light.

- Allow one to enclose you in a pillar of light which will then dissolve into cascading light beams, like cascading golden sequins, and fill you with radiance.

- You will find yourself sliding down the tree.

- Sit with your back to the Sun tree and let the light continue to enter your Crown through the leaves.

- Afterwards if you are very athletic and have a strong tree, you might like to climb into the branches, and connect with the shaman on the cosmic tree, but do be careful.

Affirmation

'I am one, I am all, all is one' is the affirmation of the Crown chakra.

Working with the Crown chakra

Mysticism is defined as an overwhelming sense of being in complete unity or oneness with the deity or cosmos, whether this is interpreted as a unity with God, the Goddess, with Nature, or the Buddhist undifferentiated state of bliss, Nirvana.

Mystical experiences are inevitably personal and, though the state in which a mystical experience occurs may be reached through years of contemplation, study and aestheticism, the experience, which may be a single moment of enlightenment or a series of visions, is invariably spontaneous.

The US psychologist Abraham Maslow defined mysticism in terms of peak experiences, to encompass the whole spectrum of altered states of consciousness, secular as well as religious. Maslow believed we can all attain these wonderful moments when we have total understanding of the meaning of the universe and our place in it, when the whole jigsaw comes together, even if seconds later we drop it. Though such moments are by their nature spontaneous, certain situations can trigger them. I have suggested a few from my own research.

- Sit on a sunny shore or by a fountain in sunlight looking at the rippling water and allowing the sound to fill your mind. I once saw a rainbow right in the centre of the fountain.

- Touch the soft cheek of a baby or watch him or her in sleep and know that we are one with the heart of innocence and beauty.

- Make love at an ancient site or on the seashore under a Full Moon or in newly mown grass with someone with whom you share spiritual as well as physical love, and merge as one flesh and spirit.

- Listen to a choir, especially singing Gregorian chants in a cathedral as sunset filters through the windows.

- Walk or dance a labyrinth, for example the one in Chartres Cathedral or one of the tiled ones that are appearing in cathedrals and churches throughout the world as this ancient form of spiritualism is revived. There is a copy of the labyrinth at Chartres in Grace Cathedral in San Francisco. Find one of the turf labyrinths or even a maze and surrender yourself to the green pathways.

- Watch the dawn rise over a standing stone on Midsummer's Day (there are many that are accessible to the public and rarely visited), knowing you are one with those who over the millennia also witnessed the dance of the Sun.

- Go into a museum in the early morning, one where you are allowed to hold Roman pottery or touch the statues. Again allow yourself to become one with the ancient world.

- Lie on the grass in the darkness and look up at the stars, focusing on one point and letting the others merge and dance so that the Milky Way does flow like a river of star milk.

- Run downhill in a fierce wind, ride a horse at full speed along sand or through the desert, roll in snow, swim underwater among shoals of fish or even through the illuminations of the pool lights at your local swimming baths.

As your Crown chakra becomes more efficient through use, so these experiences will increase and occur when you least expect them. Gradually the vibrations of your life will increase so that the mundane is tinged with magic and you do walk through the stars in the city streets.

TEN

Healing, Cleansing and Empowering the Chakras

As you work with the individual chakras, so their self-regulating mechanism becomes more efficient and the negativity and pollution of everyday life are more easily filtered out. But it is hard to have a peak experience or to connect with the divine core in everything if your upstairs neighbour drums all night long or you are worried about how you will pay the bills or cope with a child or partner in crisis. The negative thought forms representing the reaction to noise, traffic congestion and overcrowding created by people living in a city, hang over it like a smog and inevitably filter through the aura into the chakras.

In such a case, our spiritual as well as physical immune system is gradually eroded, our chakras get clogged with the pressures and actual pollution of daily life and our auras get darker or duller. Eventually the dis-ease may be manifest in the physical body as a migraine or a stomach upset, an inability to relax or insomnia.

Emotional crises too may cause us to put blocks on the negative sensations, to blot out pain or unhappiness and so we unwittingly contribute to the blocking process of the chakras.

Balancing the chakra system

Regular cleansing and strengthening of the chakras will remove these blockages and restore balance to the chakra system. Though this chapter is primarily about healing oneself, the methods can, like those in the following two chapters, be applied to the professional therapeutic situation.

Since all the chakras are connected, it makes sense to work with the entire chakra system and, unless you have a relatively stress-free life, to use the methods I have suggested for harmonising the chakras once a week or whenever you feel that life is becoming too much or your muscles warn you of tension.

Then, if there are any special problems physically, mentally or spiritually (usually all three are intricately entwined) that are related to a particular chakra, you can use one of the healing methods on pages 134–137 or the ways I suggest in this chapter for specific chakra healing.

You cannot infuse too much healing energy as, when the system is back in harmony, the energies automatically switch off, just as when you are charging your mobile phone, once it is full of power it does not keep absorbing it ad infinitum. Once we unclog the chakra system, the wondrous self-regulating system is able to operate efficiently once more.

As I have said many times in this book because it is so crucial, trust your psyche and your hands to guide you and become a channel through which Earth and cosmic energies flow.

Trees such as the oak and yew live for more than a thousand years simply by being open to the natural energy sources.

Using crystals

Crystals are without doubt the most potent but also gentle method of chakra cleansing and empowering, and the following method is one you can use either for yourself or on anyone you are healing. I have listed the crystals for each chakra again here, so that you do not need to refer back to earlier chapters. If an area of your body is painful, tense or slow to heal you can add a second crystal or even a ring of four or five at the appropriate chakra. If you are not sure of the source of the problem, use your pendulum (see page 11) or allow your mind to go blank and let your hand guide you.

Root chakra	Bloodstone, garnet, red jasper, lodestone, obsidian, smoky quartz, ruby and black tourmaline.
Sacral chakra	Banded orange agate, amber, aquamarine, orange calcite, carnelian, coral, fluorite, moonstone and rutilated quartz.
Solar Plexus chakra	Golden beryl, yellow calcite, citrine, desert rose, tiger's eye and topaz.
Heart chakra	Moss agate, aventurine, green calcite, emerald, jade, kunzite, rose quartz and green tourmaline.
Throat chakra	Blue lace agate, blue beryl, lapis lazuli, blue quartz, sapphire and turquoise.
Brow chakra	Amethyst, azurite, kunzite, lapis lazuli, sodalite and sugilite.
Crown chakra	White and purple banded amethyst, diamond, pearl, crystal quartz, and brilliant purple sugilite.

Cleansing, balancing and empowering the chakras

All three functions are inextricably linked in this method, which, by using the appropriate crystal/s on each of the chakras at the same time, allows the individual energy system to draw on both Earth and cosmic powers to restore harmony to the whole system. This in turn will restore light to the aura. Crystals are living energies that are perfectly balanced and so can restore harmony to your chakras faster than any other method.

- Before starting this ritual, soak a small, clear crystal quartz and an amethyst in a bowl of water for eight hours.

- Select three or four crystals for each chakra, choosing flat crystals, rather than rounded, about the size of a medium coin.

- Place your chakra crystals in a large crystal or ceramic dish.

- Sprinkle around the dish a circle of sea salt for the Earth element, saying:

  Bless and protect, healing flow, sorrow go.

- Light a sandalwood or frankincense incense stick and make a clockwise circle of smoke just outside the salt circle, repeating the chant.

- Stand the incense in a tall container or incense burner where it can burn safely.

- Next light a purple candle and make a circle of fire around the circle of salt and incense, again reciting the chant. Place the candle somewhere that it can burn safely.

- Finally sprinkle some of the water in which you had previously soaked the crystal quartz and amethyst, directly on to the circle of salt, saying the words for the final time.

- Keep the remaining water to hand for use later.

- You have now created a triple circle of power and protection. By using the substances that represent the four ancient elements, you have combined the energies to make the quintessence or ether, the highest vibrational level of the spirit. This is the level at which we can draw down the higher healing energies to help us in healing, whether of ourselves or others.

- You must now choose the crystals to be used on each chakra. Start with the Root chakra, for which you will need a minimum of two crystals, as you will be placing one on each foot.

- Hold the index finger of your power hand, the one you write with, over the dish.

- You may prefer to use your pendulum instead of your finger.

- You will feel a vibration in your finger (or pendulum) over the correct crystal. If the vibrating continues, allow it to select a second or even a third crystal even if you were not consciously aware of a problem with that specific chakra.

- When the vibrating ceases, plunge your finger (or pendulum) into the crystalline water you used in creating the circle and shake it dry, before choosing the next crystal/s.

- Continue until you have crystals for all seven chakras.

- Lie on a bed or comfortable couch.

- Place a chakra crystal on each of the seven main chakras of your body (see diagram).

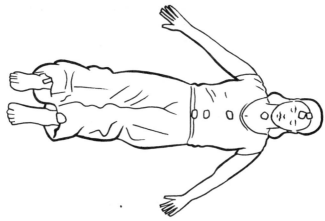

Lying with crystals on the feet (for the Root chakra) and on the Sacral, Solar Plexus, Heart, Throat, Brow and Crown chakras

- It is slightly easier if someone else places the crystals, but it is quite possible to do it yourself if you begin at the feet and position the Brow and Crown chakra crystals when you are lying down. If necessary, you can use a little tape to secure them.
- If you are healing others, play soft music and create a scene with words as you place the crystals.
- For the Root chakra, place a dark red or brown crystal on each ankle.
- For the Sacral chakra, place the orange crystal on your womb or genitals.
- Place the yellow Solar Plexus crystal just above your navel or between the navel and the chest.
- The green Heart chakra crystal should be in the centre of your chest or between your breasts, level with your heart.
- The blue Throat crystal is set around the Adam's apple.
- The indigo/purple Brow crystal should be on the centre of the brow just above the eyes.
- Finally the clear quartz or violet Crown crystal should be on your hairline in the centre.
- Do not worry about visualising the energies. Close your eyes and allow the colours to swirl upwards and downwards, merging and forming rainbow light beams. You may feel warm and even drift in and out of sleep.

- When you can feel gentle humming vibrations within you like a well-tuned engine or a flight of bees circling around flowers, slowly remove the crystals one by one and drop them into the crystalline water.

- Look into the mirror and you will see psychically or with your physical eyes that the area around your head appears quite luminous.

- Gaze at each crystal and words will come to mind about crystal fountains, rainbows, flowing waters and warm sunlit grass, waterfalls and a gentle sea.

- Continue to weave scenes until you naturally fall into silence.

- Afterwards *read* the aura and note any areas that may need ongoing care. These may be due to the energy showing signs of depletion or over activity at specific chakra points.

- If there are any areas of discomfort or pain or which you know need special attention, circle the relevant chakra with its own crystal, allowing your hand to direct it anti-clockwise and clockwise in turn, following the energies you *feel* in the chakra itself.

Using chakra fragrances

I first used this method when working with the aura but it is equally effective to cleanse, balance and empower the chakras directly since both are gateways to the same energy source. Each chakra/auric level has an associated fragrance that can be evoked either in incense or as an oil. Certain fragrances, however, do seem especially potent for directly influencing the chakras and so I have modified the fragrances that I had used for a number of years in aura work, as a result of research I recently carried out while in Sweden.

In the chapters on the individual chakras I said that you could increase the energy flowing through a particular chakra and remove any stagnation or blockage by burning particular fragrances. This is most effective for the Heart chakra because its natural element, Air, rules oils and incenses. This is also a good method of instantly strengthening any chakra whose qualities you will need at a specific time, for example burning fennel or lemongrass to stimulate the Throat chakra if you need to communicate clearly but with compassion. This would also be good if you were surrounded by a lot of spite, gossip and backbiting and would soften the words of all present, even if they were operating at a lower level of chakra in their own lives.

Using incenses or herbs

As with the crystals, I have listed the herbs and incenses again here, so that you do not need to refer back to earlier in the book. The lists, however, do not correspond directly with those in the chakra chapters because I have listed those herbs that work particularly well as incense or smudge and concentrated on those that are especially effective in healing.

During pregnancy, you should avoid basil, bay, clary sage, cypress, dragon's blood, fennel, mistletoe, myrrh, peppermint, rosemary, sage, thyme and wintergreen. Check with a herbalist or pharmacist if you are pregnant, and avoid all smoke magic at least for the first three months, and possibly for the whole pregnancy. If you suffer from any chronic medical condition, again check with a pharmacist before using incenses, oils or herbs, as rosemary, for example, is bad for high blood pressure and heart problems. The aforementioned list of herbs to avoid is not comprehensive and refers only to fragrances I have mentioned in this book.

Root chakra / Etheric layer	Basil, cypress, ivy, mimosa, patchouli, tea tree and vetivert.
Sacral chakra / Emotional layer	Clary sage, jasmine, lemon balm, lotus, myrrh, rosewood and ylang-ylang.
Solar Plexus chakra / Mental layer	Cinnamon, copal, dragon's blood, juniper, lemon, rosemary and pine.
Heart chakra / Astral layer	Geranium, hyacinth, lilac, mugwort, rose, strawberry, vanilla and vervain.
Throat chakra / Etheric template	Fennel, ferns, lavender, lemongrass, lemon verbena and peppermint.
Brow chakra / Celestial body	Mistletoe, sage, sandalwood, sweetgrass and thyme.
Crown chakra / Ketheric template	Bay, benzoin, chamomile, frankincense, gum Arabic (acacia), juniper, desert and mountain sage (sage brush), orange and rosemary.

If you want to increase the general transference of energy throughout the entire chakra system, you can surround yourself with seven different chakra fragrances. Incense tends to be safer for this ritual, though oil is fine to burn in a room where you are absorbing energy over a time or influencing others. This ritual is especially effective in sunlight. You can use it to balance the chakras of other people. As they lie with their eyes closed, weave images of the different fragrances, for example of lemon trees under a brilliant Mediterranean blue sky or tall pine trees blowing in the wind.

- You can work outdoors in a sheltered spot. Use special garden incense that is easily obtainable.

- Alternatively if you have a large garden or a balcony with enough room, use pots of the actual herbs to surround you.

- If you are using incense, one stick of each variety in each container should be sufficient.

- Make sure the incense sticks are in a deep, upright container. You can improvise with jars, cans or bottles if you run out of holders, or, if you are outdoors you can set them in soil or pottery plant pots. Always ensure that they are at a safe distance from yourself and any fabrics.

- Lie facing north on cushions, a sofa or a bed. You may choose to lie on the floor, or if outdoors, you may lie on grass or even in a sheltered spot on sand near the sea.

- To the south of your head place a Crown chakra incense stick such as frankincense.

- At Brow level on either side of you place a Brow chakra incense. Place the appropriate chakra incense level with your Throat chakra on both sides of your neck, with your Heart chakra on both sides, for the Solar

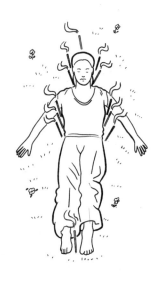

Plexus above your navel on both sides, and level with your womb or genitals for the Sacral chakra. Finally to the north of your feet place a single Root chakra incense.

- Close your eyes and visualise the smoke as different colours, swirling in bands both within and beyond your body in the auric field around you, spiralling upwards and downwards converging and filling you with radiant colour.
- You may see your body as a rainbow.
- Wait until the incense is burned through and use the time to weave dreams and allow images and sounds to form that may speak of events to come or possible pathways you might follow.

Using candles

You can carry out the same ritual using small a circle of twelve coloured candles in broad-based holders or metal trays. Each will be approximately 30 degrees apart. This ritual is especially magical when carried out in full moonlight either indoors with the window open if warm enough or outdoors in a sheltered spot where there is no risk of causing a fire.

- Make sure the circle is large enough that you can sit in the centre and be at a safe distance from the candles.
- You will need one candle each for the Root chakra (red) and Crown chakra (violet, white or gold). You will then need two candles each for the five remaining chakras: Sacral (orange), Solar Plexus (yellow), Heart (green or pink), Throat (blue) and Brow (indigo).
- Position the red Root chakra candle first to the north of the circle.
- Arrange the Sacral chakra candles to the east and west of the Root candle, moving southwards. Then position the Solar Plexus candles next to each Sacral chakra candle in the east and west of the circle, again moving southwards.
- Place the two Heart chakra candles on either side of the circle, then the Throat candles and the two Brow candles.
- Complete the circle with the single violet, white or gold candle in the south to represent the Crown chakra.
- Light the red Root chakra candle first.
- Then light each of the candles in ascending chakra order: for example, the Sacral candle on the east side of the circle, then the one in the west, followed by the eastern Solar Plexus and so on.

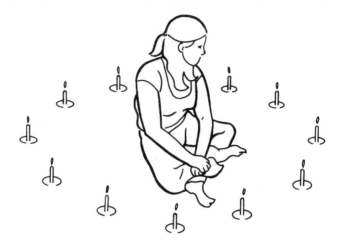

- Blow out the taper and sit inside the circle facing the Crown chakra candle.

- Allow the coloured energies to enter your mind. If it helps, inhale slowly and gently through your nose, hold your breath for a count of three and gently exhale through your mouth.

- When you can feel the buzzing sensation, you know the healing is complete. You can then blow out the candles in the order of lighting, sending healing to whoever needs it.

- If you are carrying out the healing for someone else, sit to the north of the Root candle outside the circle facing inwards so you can see all the candles and the person you are healing.

- Allow a gentle colour visualisation to come and describe what you see and feel. Do not try to think of the right words; they will come. As a bonus, you will find your own chakras become harmonious as you are filled with rhythmic power.

- When your own increased harmony indicates to you that the healing is complete, ask your subject to blow out the candles and send the light to her/himself and to whoever needs it.

Healing with higher energies

The aforementioned three methods and those on pages 134–139 can be used from the beginning of your own chakra exploration. However, once you have carried out at least some work on the Heart chakra, you will discover that, since this is a gateway chakra, you can channel energy via the higher chakras from angelic and cosmic forces as pure light. You can use this method both for self-healing of your own chakra system or specific chakras and for healing the chakras of others.

This is a very special method of healing and if you have not attempted the exercise on page 94 for contacting your special angel, read it through now. Use the love in your Heart chakra to ask, in your own words, that you may be used as a vehicle for light and healing.

- Work in sunlight or by golden candlelight and have crystals and plants or flowers in each of the main chakra colours, plus fruits, seeds and uncooked vegetables also in the seven colours to increase the natural flow of the life force or *prana*.

- In preparation for the end of the ritual, soak a small, clear crystal quartz and an amethyst in a bowl of water for eight hours.

- Make an arc with your hands and hold your fingers up to the light. Visualise an angelic force or radiant light transmitting pure gold and white liquid power through the Crown of your head. This should then flow down through your Brow, spiralling as it reaches each chakra, down through the Throat chakra, into the Heart and thereby through your arms to your fingers. Remember the Heart chakra rules the minor chakras in the palms of the hands.

- At the same time, the light will be entering your outstretched fingertips. You may be aware of tingling or faint golden sparks.

- Flow with the energy.

- To heal and harmonise the entire chakra system, move your hands from the Crown chakra to the Root, working with each chakra in turn. At each chakra, hold your hands for about a minute, or for longer if you feel the need. Be guided by the flow and not the clock.

- You may return later to any chakra that seems to need extra healing or untangling.

- Hold your two hands facing downwards and close together, fingers pointing downwards, about three finger-breadths above the anterior fontanelle of yourself or the person you are healing (see diagram on page 104).

- You do not need to do anything, merely allow the light to flow downwards, inwards and flow in and around the Crown chakra, clearing, harmonising and empowering.

- Next hold your hands 2–3 cm (1 in) from the eyes as though covering the eyes. Feel the light flowing into and around the Brow chakra. You will identify the centre by the whirlpool sensation but, if you wait, the energies will emerge and continue to flow (see diagram on page 90).

- Move downwards to the Throat chakra. Cross your hands over the centre of the throat or hold your hands about 2 cm (1 in) from the throat on either side, fingers pointing downwards (see diagram on page 78).

- Move next down to the Heart chakra and again cross your hands, this time over the centre of the breast or chest, 2–3 cm (1 in) away from the body (see diagram on page 65).

- Continue to feel the light flowing.

- Once the channel is open, light will flow until you have completed healing.

- Carrying out this form of healing for another person will not deplete your own strength, rather increase your own chakra power and harmony.

- Direct your hands now towards the Solar Plexus chakra, with your fingers still pointing downwards and not touching the body, around the waist and between the navel and the chest so that your hands almost touch. You can identify the centre by the mini-whirlpool sensation (see diagram on page 54).

- Next point your hands downwards to form a 'v' just below the navel towards the Sacral chakra. Here the energies of the two hands will merge and form a single beam of healing light (see diagram on page 43).

- At this point, sit down, cross your legs and raise first your left and then your right foot, or ask your subject to do this.

- Cupping your hands around the sole, the minor chakra point through which you can most easily access the Root chakra, allow the energies to flow and rise to warm the base of the spine and perineum area.

- Return to any chakras that need attention, thank the angels and wise guides or the power of light that has filled you with healing and plunge your hands into the water in which the amethyst and crystal quartz have been soaked.

- Shake your hands and you will be rewarded with shimmering light beams.

Some practitioners prefer to make actual contact between hands and skin both when healing the chakras of themselves and others. This can be very powerful in cases of chronic exhaustion, illness or depression. If you do not know the person well, make certain they will not feel threatened by such close contact and spend time talking gently to establish a spiritual rapport (see the next chapter for healing friends and relations).

Be aware also that such healing can lead to emotional bonds growing between you and the subject. Unless you are to be involved in long-term care, take time to move out of the joint personal space by moving once more down through the chakras, but this time with your hands about 5 cm (2 in) away. Also direct the subject's positive feelings towards close friends and family, perhaps to repairing a relationship.

ELEVEN

Chakras
and Relationships

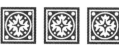

Just as chakras regulate our internal system, so they are also part of a chakra system that connects people, especially in close relationships. Ties grow up that can be seen or sensed clairvoyantly as bands of colour extending between the chakras of two or more people. These ties develop between parents, children, siblings, friends, even colleagues with whom you have a great deal of contact over a prolonged period.

The links tend to be more enduring than those reflected purely in the colour of the aura as this can be affected by temporary mood swings or current events. This is especially so when studying a group of people and can reveal the bonds between chakras and the nature of those links.

Understanding the links

At their best, chakra connections offer a secure mutual support system and in times of challenge or crisis can strengthen the people so linked. A child, for example, will have very strong initial bonds especially with the mother. It is these links that account for telepathic connections.

Of course, these chakra bonds vary in intensity at different stages in the life cycle. As the world outside the home expands for a teenager, he or she will extend chakra tentacles in a variety of directions. At the same time, links with parents and immediate family, especially those emanating from the Solar Plexus or centre of personal power, will become more slender. Sacral connections can blossom with emerging sexuality.

Grandchildren create new bright strands from the Heart. In contrast, when a relation or close friend dies, the sudden severing can be reflected as a general loss of colour throughout the whole system for many months.

When there is discoloration, blockage or a partial fracture in a chakra strand between family members, there may be unresolved relationship issues. In a prime relationship, for example between parent and adult child, this can adversely affect the individuals for years or even a lifetime, making other relationships difficult. (See the next chapter for the chakra links between couples.)

Identifying the problem chakra areas and healing these will result in a freeing of energies and improvement on every level. For though most blockages originate in the lower three or personal chakras, the Root, Sacral and Solar Plexus, their effects can prevent the individuals from functioning well at the higher levels and breaking the patterns that can hold them back.

Chakra readings to identify the ties

Begin by studying pairs or groups of people with whom there are obvious connections, for example a mother and baby or young child. You will probably observe a strong bond between the Root and Sacral chakras and a pink or green band between the Heart levels. If the mother is depressed or anxious, there may be discoloration or even fractures in the links, but they will nevertheless be there and this is a case for offering practical help or support as well as chakra healing work (see page 134).

Continue to practise informally at family gatherings or with groups of friends, again looking at the space between the people at the different chakra levels.

Begin first at the level of the top of the head. Close your eyes, open them, blink and then observe if there is a link and, if so, if it is like a thick cord or if there are any tangles or even breaks.

Continue until you have studied all seven chakra areas. You may see the connections externally or in your mind's eye. Both are equally valid.

Do not be surprised if some people have few or no connections. A jovial uncle may be projecting bonhomie as a shield for his true solitary nature and the responses of others may not be reaching him. A possessive parent may be connected by the Sacral chakra of personal need for self-esteem to the Solar Plexus or Heart chakra of a grown-up child. The link may be destructive as perhaps the child seeks to disentangle.

Recording your findings

As you become more practised you may find it helpful to keep a record of your observations so that you can study a variety of interconnections.

Unless you are working with people as part of a healing/diagnostic session, you will need to be tactful about the way you record. However, diagrams need only be small and you can easily recall what you saw by closing your eyes when you are alone and quiet, and allowing the earlier observations to re-form in your mind's eye.

Draw outlines of the people you observed and then, using coloured crayons as you did for marking auras (see page 23), draw the individual chakras and the lines between them. Note that these may change colour part way through.

Mark the tangles and fractures and any area where the colour fades or is unduly harsh, indicating an excess of energy, usually from one side.

In time you will recognise and work with the chakra connections of a whole family or social group.

Interpreting your readings

Re-read the chapters on the individual chakras to remind yourself of the emotional and spiritual significance of each chakra colour and its lack or excess.

Then begin by studying the lines that you have drawn between an individual and either one particular person or other members of the group.

A key link is between the Throat chakras. If this is clear, usually blue, then there is good communication between the people, trust and honesty. Tangles, discoloration, fractures or an absence of links will be mirrored and caused by problems in the three lower, personal chakras, Root, Sacral and Solar Plexus. You may find tentacles from the lower chakras of one or more people; for example, power struggles from the Solar Plexus chakras or, more usually, needs and possessiveness from the Sacral chakra or suppressed anger from the Root.

If the relationship is good, you may find an indigo clear telepathic bond at the Brow level and this will be especially strong between a mother and child of any age, but may be present in other relationships with a close emotional bond. Watch out for darkness coming from one of the lower chakras to the Brow of another, as this can be an unconscious form of psychic attack, where suppressed resentments or frustrated emotions from the bottom two chakras have become transformed into negative energy.

Occasionally you may get a Crown chakra link especially in relationships where one person has been a willing care giver to someone who is sick or disabled, though this may be clouded if the care giver is unsupported.

Rich green or pink strands from the Heart chakras indicate a deep and very healthy relationship, free from the possessiveness or need for constant reassurance from the Sacral chakras or self-interest from the Solar Plexus. This characterises a deep friendship or creative family relationship. Links with the lower chakras of another indicate that one party may care rather more deeply than the other. If the colour becomes murky, one party may be extending possessive tentacles to feed his or her own inadequacy.

If in doubt, study the chakra colours of the individuals to see the source of any negativity.

Clear yellow Solar Plexus links indicate that the relationship is one in which all parties can maintain their own identity and is creative on a mental and intellectual as well as emotional level. This is a connection often found in colleagues who have worked together well for a time and there may be Heart links. Watch out for lower chakra links between colleagues, especially if these are entwined with the Solar Plexus chakra. While they may lead to more permanent attachments in personal life, clouded or fractured links can indicate a potential office affair. This may not be good for the well-being of the workplace, especially if the person has Root, Sacral or Heart ties extending to a colleague rather than to a spouse.

Sacral ties in rich orange of needs and desires are very common especially between family members and cover the whole nurturing/nurtured spectrum. Only if there is darkness or tangles should you trace these links back to the chakra of the individual who is emanating the negativity or possessiveness. Sacral ties that are wound around a higher chakra indicate that emotional pressure may be holding back one or both parties.

Finally the red Root links between friends and family members indicate close domestic attachments that are entirely healthy and necessary. If there is darkness or harshness or a tangled cord, see whether one chakra is draining another of energy or if there is suppressed resentment or anger.

Healing problem areas in the relationships of others

If you are working within a therapeutic situation, you can use the methods I suggested on pages 118 and 126 to cleanse and harmonise the chakra system of your client or clients. You may choose to use candles or fragrances.

However, it is quite possible, without interfering in the dynamics of relationships between family, friends or even colleagues or infringing on their free will, to use visualisation to send healing energies to tangled or discoloured chakras without setting up a formal session. This can clear stagnation or impasses that will enable them to move on to a more creative stage in the relationship. This has a beneficial effect on all around, especially for those who may have ties to both parties, for example if they are your parents.

Do not underestimate the healing power of speech (see page 30 for chakra sound work). Often those close to us welcome time, perhaps sitting by candlelight on a quiet evening or during a daytime walk by the sea or in the countryside, to unburden their hearts and talk through problems with a loving third person who will not apportion blame nor take sides.

If indoors, you could burn oils and incenses associated with individual chakras that may need attention (see the separate chakra entries for these).

Using the healing power of light

This method is good for healing family relationships or those of close friends, including your own relationship with someone who is not present. (See also pages 136–137.)

• Work in brilliant sun or full moonlight or surrounded by a circle of alternate gold and silver candles if it is dark.

- Use the diagrams you drew of two or more people in your family group and their chakra connections and place it within a pool of light within the circle.

- Name each person and speak a few words about their positive qualities.

- Take your clear crystal pendulum and swirl it over the diagram clockwise so that rainbows of light are reflected from it on to the paper.

- Pass the pendulum first over the separate chakras, beginning at the Root and moving to the Crown of each person depicted in turn.

- Move the pendulum anti-clockwise if there is any darkness or you can feel a blockage in an individual chakra; then turn it clockwise to infuse positive energy, again reflecting the light beams through the pendulum.

- Speak encouraging words over the relevant chakra. For example, over the Heart chakra of a person who is having problems resisting the manipulative needs of an elderly relation, you might say:

    Move freely in love and return us to harmony, as and if you will.

- Then work on the chakra strands, gently untangling any knots with an anti-clockwise swing of the pendulum and healing any fractures or restoring colours with a clockwise movement. If a link is slender, do not try to build it up as it may be one that is naturally becoming less intense.

- Equally, I do not think you should cut any cords, even destructive ones, unless you are working directly with at least one of the people involved and it is requested (see page 146 for severing old redundant links).

- Finally, work on the cross-chakra links. Use a clockwise swirl of light to strengthen the chakra of the individual who is perhaps being weakened by a link. This may be indicated by paleness in their chakra and harshness in the chakra colour of the instigator of the power loss.

You can adapt this method for use in a therapeutic situation with two people, such as two or more family members.

- Sit the connected family members in sunlight, moonlight or within a candlelit circle and pass the pendulum over the chakras and chakra connections directly, untangling and energising where necessary. This can have a very positive effect where family members or friends have reached an impasse but where there is an underlying well of positive emotions. It can be especially helpful if you weave words of love, healing and harmony as you work with the different colours.

Studying your own interactions

Once you are familiar with chakra interpretation, you can work on the dynamics of your own place in a family, social or work relationship. Work if possible in soft candlelight or as the sunset floods the sky.

- Stand side-on, facing the other person in front of a mirror.

- Again, half-close your eyes and, beginning first at the level of the top of the head, close your eyes, open them, blink and then see if there is a link. If there is, is it like a thick cord or are there any tangles, or even breaks?

- Continue until you have studied all seven chakra areas.

- Draw two outlines and colour in the strands you observe, marking in any knots, areas of darkness or breaks in the strands.

- You can ask the other person to draw his or her own lines of connections on to another diagram The two drawings are often remarkably similar and even a beginner can identify connections intuitively. (See the next chapter for interconnections between you and a lover or permanent love partner.)

Sensing the connections

If you find it difficult to relax into using clairvoyance, especially when studying your own interactions, you can use a pendulum for clairsentience (literally clear-sensing), and then combine this with the method above for healing and do away with the need for a diagram at all.

- Pass a crystal pendulum slowly between the chakras of you and the person to whom you are emotionally linked.

- You will find the pendulum will move in clockwise circles or ellipses if the link is present, but will not move if there is no connection or if there is a break in the thread. Tangles are usually felt as anti-clockwise swirling or a dragging sensation, like being caught in a knotted thread.

- Now move the pendulum diagonally in the space between you to trace chakra links on different levels.

- You can heal any problems as you find them, using light reflected through the pendulum, amplified by candles if necessary.

- If the other person is absent, make your mind blank, allowing an image of yourself and your friend or relation to build up with coloured lights between the relevant chakras. Afterwards draw your impressions and heal using the diagram method.

Healing your family chakra links

Using mutual smudging

I suggested smudging in the Crown chakra chapter as a way of finding your still centre. It is also a powerful way of working with a friend or family member to cleanse the chakras and their connections and, at the same time, to empower the relationship.

- Use sage or cedar smudge sticks. These can be easily obtained either from a New Age store or by mail order. Alternatively they can be made by binding three or four fronds of pine about 23 cm (9 in) long tightly together at regular intervals with non-flammable twine and leaving them to dry but not go brown. You could also use large, firm incense sticks in sage, rosemary, juniper, cedar or pine, all of which are cleansing (see also page 123).

- Light the tip of your own and then the other person's stick from a beeswax or pure white candle and blow out the flame so the tip is glowing and there is a steady stream of smoke.

- Leave the candle in a broad holder close by. You can use it to relight the smudge stick during the ritual if necessary.

- Face each other about 10 cm (4 in) apart, as though you were going to dance, and, beginning at each other's Crown chakra, spiral the sticks first anti-clockwise and then clockwise around the chakra and then in the space between you, moving in unison. You may find as you smudge each chakra connection that the two smudge sticks form a spiralling pattern between you.

- You can create a joint chant that you repeat faster and faster as you move rhythmically. For example:

    Father Sky, Mother Earth, cleanse, empower, new life give birth.

    Joined we are in love not need, in mutual joy all anger freed.

- Continue to work down the chakras in the same way until you smudge around the other person's base of the spine and finally feet, for the Root chakra, making a downward sweep with the smudge to link to the Earth power and repeating:

    Mother Earth, new life give birth.

- Move up the other person's chakras and the chakra links again, first anti-clockwise then clockwise, and finish the ritual by raising the smudge over the head of the other to the sky, calling out to release the power:

  Father Sky, accept our cry.

- Sink to the ground and exchange the smudge sticks. Then gently extinguish them either in a bowl of sand or the earth if you are working outdoors, saying:

  So banish sadness, linger only gladness.

- Take the candle and place it between you as you sit.

- On the candle, mark one notch 1 cm (½ in) down from the flame and a second notch 1 cm (½ in) below that. Allow the other person to speak, remaining silent until the candle is burned to the first notch. Any lingering bitterness will give way to gentler words and, when it is your turn to talk, try to maintain the softer tone, speaking healing from the heart and allowing new strands to grow.

- If there are any really difficult issues, after your candle time, take turns to burn dark threads into the candle flame, letting any residual anger or resentment burn away in the flame.

- Afterwards, sit quietly holding hands and, when you are ready, blow out the flame, sending the light to each other.

If you prefer a quieter ritual, place a bowl of desert or mountain sage in a flat ceramic bowl between you and sit and smudge each other's chakras and their links with a feather or your hand, perhaps playing gentle music instead of chanting.

TWELVE

Chakras, Love and Sexuality

With lovers and permanent partners, the chakra links are even stronger than with other family members because the additional power of sexual attraction can form the basis for profound spiritual connection. For when you combine your individual chakra systems into one during an act of lovemaking, you are opening your souls, your innermost beings to one another.

The links of love

Other than lovemaking, there are other non-sexual levels that are equally important in creating the rich interconnection and mutual support system of positively entwined chakras. This evolves over a period of years as a result of joint emotions and positive shared experiences, for example childbirth, children, holidays, mutual interests and dreams, the same sense of humour, perhaps even past-life connections. These roots can be strengthened through chakra sex and through other mutual chakra work, such as massage. In this way, channels can be formed through which everyday differences and difficulties can be resolved on a level far deeper than words.

Increased harmony can also be attained by cutting external negative chakra ties that divert energy from the relationship. These can be ongoing conflicts of loyalty, perhaps children at a demanding stage on their own life path, hostile relations, ex-partners, friends who resent your closeness or demanding work colleagues. If either of you have suffered betrayal or rejection in earlier relationships, guilt and regrets can spill over into your present relationship, even if the hurt occurred ten or more years before. You may be aware of an area that acts as a flashpoint even on the sunniest day or at the most relaxed moment.

As a result of positive chakra work together, these external redundant influences or pressures that choke the free flow of the lower chakras do become less invasive. Communication will become more honest and you will experience increased connection at the higher chakra levels.

Tracing the connections

Love at first sight begins with eye contact, whether across a crowded room or on the early morning commuter train. The Brow chakras make a connection and any psychic links, whether from past lives or present, create a feeling that you have known the other person for years.

This is even before the Root chakra 'find a mate' magnetism (much-loved by anthropologists and zoologists) is activated. At this psychic level, either the separate auras open and interconnect or one or the other denies access. Before long, if all goes well, this chakra will be in overdrive and you will be picking up the phone at the same moment and finding you both went on holiday as children to the same part of the coast many miles from where you now live.

Next, the Throat chakra makes a connection; blushing and stammering can result from this normally well-organised centre being flooded with emotions from the lower chakras. The Root recognises a kindred nest-builder and compatible gene source, the Sacral is sexually and emotionally aroused as the affirmation of desirability by another boosts self-worth, while the Solar Plexus is trying to match the initial information on the mental compatibility score sheet.

The Heart chakra is filtering all these messages and at the same time responding to a deep awareness that the embryo relationship may have sufficient potential to reach the golden wedding stage and beyond.

Finally, the Crown chakra creates a spiritual link that in couples who remain together over decades becomes the most enduring, transcending everyday problems and ageing – and perhaps even death itself.

Of course, all these tendrils may actually grow much more gradually than this love-at-first-sight scenario. Alternatively, lust at first sight kindled at the office coffee machine may instigate an initial Root/Sacral bond; friendship and mutual interest equally might involve the Heart and Solar Plexus very early in the encounter.

Because these connections do root deep within lovers and tend to exist at most chakra points, it is inevitable that any break-up – even an amicable one – is painful. At one extreme, people who have been married for many years can pine away when a lifetime mate dies. On page 146 I have described a way of severing the tendrils between you and an ex-lover so that you are free to move on without bitterness, but you may need to repeat the ritual many times.

Working with the love relationships of others

You can carry out joint chakra readings with couples that come to see you informally or professionally for counselling and healing, but you need tremendous tact, especially if you see strong roots going from one of the couple to an absent third party. In such a case, it can be helpful to suggest separate healing sessions in which each person can voice any individual concerns. Afterwards you can work with both people to untangle any chakra knots.

- Seat the couple either side of you, facing each other.
- Have your drawing materials ready.
- Working on a diagram of the outlines of the couple, colour in the strands and the chakras, marking in any knots, areas of darkness or breaks in the strands.
- It may be helpful to create before-and-after healing diagrams, so you can recommend work at home to continue and personalise the healing process between sessions.

Interpreting your findings

Strong and clear connections at a number of chakra points and brightly coloured luminous chakras in the individuals indicate that the couple are close on a number of levels and that these bonds are mutually enriching and in no way stifling.

One link may be especially strong and, if this is at the Heart chakra, the relationship should weather almost any problems and will be deep, lasting and one that transcends sentiment, enriching all who are touched by it. The couple will make wise parents and grandparents.

Strong and clear links at Brow and Crown may indicate past-world connections and certainly confirm a telepathic bond that can transcend time and distance.

A clear Throat chakra link shows clear communication and fidelity.

Solar Plexus links, especially if accompanied by clear Heart links, demonstrate that the couple have strong separate identities that come together creatively and are intellectually as well as emotionally compatible. They make good work partners as well as lovers.

Sacral links indicate ongoing sexual attraction and a mutual satisfying of needs.

A clear, powerful Root connection indicates that the couple function well in the everyday world and are comfortable in and with their own bodies. Their home will be important to them.

If the connections link different chakras, for example, her Heart is linked to his Sacral chakra, the lower level chakra is feeding off the higher. In this case, the desires and needs of the man are more to do with gratification, rather than with the long-term altruistic love that she seeks. Inevitably there will be conflict and disappointment unless he is able to progress to a higher level of functioning. Neither is wrong or selfish, merely seeking different things from the relationship. Some relationships function in this way for many years, given compromise and acceptance. In the earlier stages of a relationship there is usually cross-chakra linking as the two individuals learn to mesh.

If there is a mass of tangles, you may find that the ends of the knots seem to connect with outside sources. These may be putting pressure on the relationship and a lot of work will be required to clear a space in which the relationship can function more effectively.

If there are no chakra connections, not even tangled ones, then the relationship is one based on two individuals who share a home, perhaps for convenience or family reasons. There may be strong strands going in other directions, indicating that their main connections are with different people. This may not necessarily mean that one of the partners is seeking love elsewhere, although strong Sacral and Heart strands going outwards to the same third source may indicate strong sexual emotions being diverted.

Often one of the couple is reaching out towards the other but these connections are ending in mid-air. If you look carefully, you may see threads very close to the other person's chakras that have faded or been cut at an earlier time and/or other strong ones extending elsewhere.

The last two situations would indicate the desirability of some separate healing work and support, especially for the rejected partner whose own chakras may be very pale as though drained of life. Indeed, if love is being dissipated into nothingness and not being replenished with energies from the other significant person, he or she may not have the energy to do anything about what is essentially a destructive situation.

Working with your own chakra connections in love

In the previous chapter, I suggested ways of identifying your chakra connections with family members and friends, and you can use similar techniques when working with a love relationship (see pages 133 and 134). If your partner is absent or unwilling to work with you, you can use the method I described on page 146. However, the following method is one that is especially effective with a partner and should be carried out at a time when you are both quiet and relaxed.

- Sit or lie facing the other and close enough to touch.

- In order to sensitise awareness of the joint energy fields surrounding you, hold your hands up to your partner's. Your palms should be about 15 cm (6 in) apart, and your fingers spread wide open.

- Close your eyes and slowly bring your hands together until they touch.

- Repeat this sequence two or three times. You may be aware of warmth and heaviness around the hands, like trying to bring the same poles of two magnets together – the closer they get, the stronger they repel each other. This is your auric field that is fuelled by your chakras and forms the ties between your chakras.

- While your hands are still sensitised, continue to work with paired hands, this time further apart, and trace the area with your hands around each of the chakras in turn, so that you each have one hand simultaneously exploring the other's chakras, beginning with the Crown and moving downwards.

- Explore the space between you on the level of each chakra and then diagonally for any cross-chakra connections. You may feel a band of energy or swirls between you and your partner's chakras.

- When you have finished, talk about what you sensed and, on a diagram of the two bodies, colour in the connections and any knots. Each of you should then colour in the other's chakras on the picture.

- You may wish to make love or lie quietly together until you fall asleep.

Healing and strengthening a relationship

There are a variety of methods you can use for healing and strengthening the chakras of your personal relationship and for helping other couples to heal their joint chakra system (see pages 134 and 137). The secret lies in two people working with their own energies. If you are helping a couple, your role therapeutically will be to advise and guide, leaving the work to be carried out privately.

Candle healing

Candle colour is very gentle and you can add crystals or mirrors to amplify the light. You can also choose scented coloured candles whose fragrances encourage gentle love and sensuality, for example lavender, sandalwood and rose. This is an extension of the candle healing I described on page 125 but the simple version can also be used, especially if the couple feel self-conscious.

This candle ritual will help to bring mutual strength and healing.

- Take seven candles in the seven main chakra colours. Use good quality, coloured candles that are the same colour all the way through (cheaper ones are usually white inside under a thin, flaky layer of dye).

- If you noticed that any chakras need special attention, you can make their candles taller or broader. Our psyches will absorb the amount of light we need.

- After dusk, create a circle of chakra colour candles: red, orange, yellow, green, blue, indigo and violet. You can substitute white for violet if you wish.

- Arrange mirrors and crystals so that the light shines in them.

- Both stand within the circle of light, side by side, lightly holding hands.

- The focus of the ritual is re-affirming the positive qualities of the relationship that may have become lost or replaced with anger, indifference or just buried beneath the pace of the modern world. However, even if your chakras and ties are strong and luminous, this ritual, carried out monthly or before a stressful period, can help to keep the energies flowing between you, and the relationship on track.

- Face first the red candle and breathe in. Gently and slowly breathe in the red light through the nose and visualise darkness being exhaled slowly through the mouth. Create your own joint breathing rhythm. Afterwards say:

    Root of power, at this hour, blessed be, joined are we.

- In each case, you can touch your partner's chakra as you speak or, if you prefer, you can continue to hold hands.
- Then speak a few words about the importance of home and domestic life.
- Face the orange candle and again breathe in orange light and exhale darkness, afterwards saying:

  Sacral power, at this hour, blessed be, joined are we.

- Then speak spontaneously on the sensual and tactile pleasures of the relationship or the conception and birth of any children, which can be very helpful in re-focusing if there have been sexual difficulties or coldness or if you are hoping for a family in the future.
- Face the yellow candle and again inhale the light and exhale darkness, afterwards saying:

  Solar power, at this hour, blessed be, joined are we.

- Then formulate aloud joint dreams and plans both immediate and long term, that you may have forgotten or been diverted from.
- Turning to the green candle, inhale green light and exhale darkness, afterwards saying:

  Heart power, at this hour, blessed be, joined are we.

- Speak of happy memories you share, of pleasures from family life and with friends and of environmental causes dear to both your hearts, anything from creating a beautiful garden at home to saving rainforests or working for cleaner seas so your descendants can bathe safely.
- Face then the blue candle, inhale blue light and exhale darkness, saying:

  Throat power, at this hour, blessed be, joined are we.

- Let words of love and reconciliation flow upwards from your heart and pledge future fidelity to each other if you feel able to at this point.
- Turn next to the indigo candle and inhale its light, exhaling darkness and say:

  Brow power, at this hour, blessed be, joined are we.

- Talk of the times you have sensed the other is sad or in danger when you are apart, recall coincidences from family life and, if you know of them, any past-life connections.

- Finally face the violet or white candle and inhale its light, exhaling any lingering darkness and say:

  Crown power, at this hour, blessed be, joined are we.

- At this point, allow your lips and heads to touch gently. Speak in your heart what it is you are not ready to say out loud or that thing to which the other person may not yet be receptive. This may be an area of the relationship where there are blind spots or difficulties that may need time and patience to resolve.

An absent partner

If your partner, or that of a client, is unwilling or uncomfortable with joint chakra work, you can map out the chakra system using a diagram of the two people involved and moving the pendulum over it. Work on joint healing with your pendulum, as described on page 134. Then, using the above ritual alone, blow out each coloured candle after you have spoken and send the light to the absent party. This can work well if you are estranged from your partner, emotionally or physically and can be repeated weekly if necessary.

Cutting ties

I have mentioned in this and the previous chapter how strands can tie us not only to other important relationships, for example children or our own parents or siblings, but to people who have moved physically from our lives, but who may evoke sorrow or guilt at a deep level that can blight present joy. Equally if you are in the middle of or have recently experienced a relationship break-up, separation or divorce, it can be helpful to cut ties with the chakras of your ex-partner.

To sever them at once or instantly would be far too painful since they are still embedded, especially if the relationship had lasted for many years or you are unwilling to let the other person go in spite of their less than loving behaviour.

You may also need to repeat the ritual many times, each time feeling a lessening of pain and connection.

This ritual is best carried out late at night.

- Take seven cords or scarves made of natural fibres in the seven main chakra colours.

- Lay them flat on a table and tie a triple knot in each in turn, beginning with the red cord and ending with violet or white, reciting:

One knot for guilt, one knot for anger,

One for lost love that makes you a stranger.

- Put the seven cords in an open box by your bed.

- On the first morning, when you wake, begin to untie the knot in the red cord, saying:

Guilt and anger stay here no longer,

Love go in peace, though now a stranger.

- Pass the red cord over the flame of a red candle, sprinkle it with salt, pass it through the smoke of a pine or frankincense incense stick and finally sprinkle a few drops of water on it, saying:

Earth, Air, Water, Fire,

Let me him/her no more desire,

Water, Fire, Earth and Air,

Home and life no longer share,

Fire, Air, Water, Earth,

Bring new life and love to birth.

- Wrap the red cord in dark silk and place it in the bottom of a drawer.

- Leave the other cords knotted in the box. For the next six mornings repeat the ritual, untying one cord at a time.

- By the seventh day you will have your seven cords wrapped in dark silk.

- Keep them for now and, if any chakra tie continues to prove painful, repeat the ritual. One day, if you are patient, you will be ready to bury the cords under a tree and let Nature begin the slow process of transforming them into new life.

Chakra sex

The most powerful way of creating positive chakra connections with a lover is through sacred sex. This involves a couple circulating joint chakra energies through their bodies, culminating in spiritual as well as physical unity in orgasm as Root and Crown chakra energies merge.

In the Tantric traditions of the East, sexual energy is used to ignite the Kundalini, the body's biological life-energy force. This resides at the base of the spine or Root chakra, and is associated with the female polarity of the Shakti or goddess energy that activates Shiva, the Sky creative force, who enters the body through the Crown chakra in the centre of the head.

This Root Shakti Earth energy is raised in lovemaking through 'riding the wave of bliss' to merge with Shiva universal energy, with the couple experiencing, through the build-up of controlled orgasmic contractions, a final cosmic orgasm. It is said that at this moment their Etheric or Spirit selves leave the body and merge on the astral plane in an evolved spiritual awareness.

Although there are many similarities, you do not need to be familiar with Tantric techniques to reach fulfilment through merging your separate chakras in lovemaking. Chakra sex is more spontaneous and has many links with westernised forms of sex magic.

You should practise sacred sex at times when you have an uninterrupted period alone together and can spend the day in quiet activities away from external pressures. Do not attempt this deep union if you are feeling temporarily resentful or cold towards the other person, because these open channels should be used only for positive emotions.

- Before chakra sex avoid the temptation to discuss any practical problems and avoid any contentious issues. If you are at home, leave the phone and faxes on answering mode, and switch off mobile phones.

- Give each other a massage using lavender or ylang-ylang essential oil, diluted as five drops of oil in 15 ml (1 tablespoon) of a carrier oil such as sweet almond. Warm the oil gently over a container of warm water.

- Use gentle circular strokes and work in turn, especially on chakra points, beginning with the head and the Crown chakra on the hairline. Work down the chakras.

- Remember, feet can be especially sensual areas and the nadis here are connected to all parts of the body. Massage the feet and the base of the spine for the Root areas, but avoid direct genital contact. Gentle circular movements on the tip of the big toe and the ankle bone are very sexually arousing.

- When you are both aroused, lie or stand so that you are not quite touching and look deeply into each other's eyes while you begin slow, gentle breathing; then touch each other lightly, still maintaining intense eye contact.

- Chakra sex works on the swingboat principle so that, with the help of your partner, you raise your energies through your chakra points to the Crown and down again to the reproductive organs (Sacral) and the perineum (Root).

- Unlike Tantric sex, you do not deliberately delay orgasm but create a rhythm whereby it builds slowly and naturally and is released spontaneously.

- You may now make contact with the coccyx, perineum, testicles, penis, the vagina and the cervix but only with feather-light touches as you are aiming to allow the sexual power to rise spontaneously through the chakras as it gathers momentum, not release it in orgasm at this point.

- The penis can now slowly enter the vagina, using slow, deep, circular movements rather than thrusts. This will circulate the energies, which are now transferred to the other person's body where they again ascend the chakras and fall like the swingboat before crossing again to the other body with increasing momentum.

- If it helps, visualise and verbalise the process as ascending light changes into the different rainbow colours and merges with the other person's chakra light in the genitals. The two columns of light are constantly changing circuits thransferred through the tongue and the skin at the chakra points.

- The light will be cascading through the body of each person through every nadir and, when it can gain no more power, at this point the chakras in both bodies will merge as, with a final upward thrust, the spirits of the couple are propelled in the pure white light out of the combined Crown chakras.

- Initially this may last only for a few moments and what can only be described as an inner firework display culminates in a physical orgasm that becomes one with the cosmic orgasm.

- In time this moment of cosmic bliss will become more prolonged, but do not force it. There may be past-life glimpses, visions of other realms, a sense of becoming one with your lover and with the cosmos, followed by a deep sense of peace as the energies subside and slowly flow back to the Root of each person.

- Lie quietly touching each other and fall gently into sleep where you may dream of the places you saw when you touched the stars.

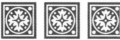

THIRTEEN

Chakras and Your Life

Chakra work and healing is not a once and for all. Even the loftiest gurus occasionally over-indulge on a packet or three of chocolate biscuits, curse as they are trapped in a traffic jam and are late for an appointment with the bank manager, or feel they are the only one home alone, unloved and unlovely on Saturday night. For the rest of us there is more stress than spirituality and we need to ascend our chakra system many, many times before it ceases to be like a game of snakes and ladders with the slippery descent waiting just as we have discovered the secrets of the universe.

Healing chakras sometimes feels more like first aid or unblocking the psychic drain system and we would sooner be slumped in front of the television in an additive-filled orgy. But even given the reality of everyday lives and pressures – and few of us can withdraw to that mountain top to meditate the golden hours away – there is a great deal we can do to prevent our chakras from becoming stagnant and depleted.

Try natural, unprocessed food and drinks that really do taste better than over-processed foods whose wrapping contains more nutrients than the contents. Spend time quietly with nature, in a wildlife garden in the city centre, on a day or weekend on a camp site in the forest or a day's bus ride into the wilderness. Make sure you get regular sleep and take gentle but ongoing exercise. Avoid x-rated films filled with horror and despair, places where there is constant loud music or over-stimulation of the senses, such as theme parks with gut-ripping rides. Cultivate friendships with people who will accept your true nature, and spend time with children and animals. Avoid over-critical relations or friends who point out our shortcomings for our own good. These are ways to restore the soul and release the chakras. This is how to allow the energies to untangle and reform spontaneously, to strengthen our sense of self-worth and well-being, and avoid the need to block our own chakras out of self-defence.

We may have to work in noisy offices or workplaces filled with machinery or technology or travel on crowded trains or on fume-filled roads. But a walk in the park at lunchtime and an after-work bath with lavender or chamomile essential oil, spending time with our garden or indoor plants, can cleanse the effects of the most stress-filled day. Use mobile phones only when necessary and ration the time spent watching television or surfing the Internet or in chat rooms that are all substitutes for face-to-face interactions or time alone cultivating inner stillness. Cook, paint, draw, dance, meditate, model with clay or wood, sing, write poetry or stories, make love with someone you love who loves you. And work with the different chakra energies at different phases of your life.

Because we are made up of pure energy we can, given the constraints of time and the demands of others create our own vibrational patterns that enable us to see the world not through rose-tinted spectacles, but with humour, compassion and a wider perspective. Walking in the rain, watching a rainbow through the window at work, digging snow or sand as we did as children, splashing in the sea or riding downhill on a bicycle. Those moments out of time that make the rest worthwhile can replenish our inner treasury and enable us to see devas, talk with angels and glimpse divinity beyond and within ourselves.

Buddhists believe we create our own chakras when we visualise or work with them and in a sense that is true, for energy is never still and the higher the vibration the less static the form. The Greek philosopher Plato described the harmony of the universe as the music of the spheres. By harmonising our own chakras over years and decades, and not just weeks or months, with the energy centres of the cosmos (think of the planets as the cosmic chakras), we can tap into an endless store of vitality and wisdom. We can heal and be healed and move in perfect harmony as we aspire to live blessed by light and Spirit.

This is a lifetime's journey that does get easier and I hope that, whether you are new to the road or an experienced traveller, this book has shared with you a few of my ideas that can act as a trigger for your own unique work and inspiration.

Useful Addresses

Chakra and energy work

Australia
The Sabian Centre
PO Box 527
Kew
Victoria 3101

UK
Caroline Shola Arewa
Inner Visions
PO Box 22032
London SW2 2WJ

USA
The Barbara Brennan School
of Healing
PO Box 2005
East Hampton
New York 11937

Candles

Australia
Price's Candles Pty Ltd
18 Gibson Avenue
Padstow
NSW 2211

UK
Price's Patent Candle Company Limited
10 York Road
London SW11 3RU

USA
Wax Wonders
221 North Main Street
Versailles
Kentucky 40383

Earth energies

Australia
Dowsers Society of New South Wales
c/o Mrs E. Miksevicius
126 Fiddens Wharf Road
Killara
New South Wales 2031

Southern Tasmania Dowsing Association
PO Box 101
Moonah
Tasmania
Australia 7009

UK
British Society of Dowsers
Sycamore Barn
Hastingleigh
Ashford
Kent TN25 5HW

Findhorn
(Workshops and courses that teach
about meditation, consciousness and
nature spirits)
Findhorn Foundation
The Park
Forres
Scotland IV36 OTS

USA
The American Society of Dowsers
Dowsers Hall
Danville
Vermont 05828 0024

Meditation, visualisation and shamanic music

Australia
New World Productions
PO Box 244 WBO
Red Hill
Queensland 4059

UK
Stress Busters
Beechwood Music
Littleton House
Littleton Road
Ashford
Middlesex TW15 1UU

USA
Raven Recordings
744 Broad Street
Room 1815
Newark
New Jersey 07102

Smudging equipment

Australia
Eartharomas Earthcraft
Magpie Flats Herb Farm
273/295 Boyle Road
Kenilworth
Queensland 4574

UK
Dreamcatcher Trading
47 Bruce Road
Sheffield
South Yorkshire S11 8QD

USA
Arizona Gateway Trading Post
Mail-HC 37
Box 919-UPS 14265
N. Hiway 93
Golden Valley AZ 86413

Spiritual healing

Australia
Australian Spiritualist Association
PO Box 248
Canterbury
New South Wales 2193

Canada
National Federation of Spiritual Healers
(Canada)
Toronto
Ontario
(Call for information 284 4798)

UK
British Alliance of Healing Associations
Mrs Jo Wallace
3 Sandy Lane
Gisleham
Lowestoft
Suffolk NR33 8EQ

National Federation of Spiritual Healers
Old Manor Farm Studio
Church Street
Sunbury on Thames
Middlesex TW16 6RG

USA
World of Light
PO Box 425
Wappingers Falls NY 12590
(Has a list of healers)

Yoga

Australia
Ananda Australia
99–107 Main Creek Road
Tanawha
Queensland 4556

UK
Yoga for Health Foundation
Ickwell Bury
Biggleswade
Bedfordshire SG18 9EF

USA
The Self-Realisation Fellowship
3880 San Rafel Avenue
Los Angeles CA 90065

Cassandra's website is
www.Cassandraeason.co.uk

Further Reading

Chakras and chakra healing

Andea, Judith, *Wheels of Light*, 1993, Bantam Books, New York

Arewa Shola, Caroline, *Opening to Spirit*, 1999, Thorsons

Brennan, Barbara Ann, *Hands of Light, A Guide to Healing Through the Human Energy Field*, 1987, Bantam Books, New York

Davies, Brenda, *The Seven Healing Chrakras*, 2000, Ulysses Press

Karagulla, Shafica and Van Gelder Kunz, Dora, *Chakras and the Human Energy Field*, 1994, Theosophical University Press

Ozaneic, Naomi, *The Elements of the Chakras*, 1989, Element

Alternative therapies

Norman, Laura, *The Reflexology Handbook*, 1998, Piatkus

Reed Gach, Michael, *Acupressure*, 1996, Piatkus

Angels

Burnham, Sophie, *A Book of Angels*, 1990, Ballantine, New York

Davidson, Gustav, *A Dictionary of Angels*, 1967, Free Press, New York

Auras

Andrews, Ted, *How to See and Read the Aura*, 1994, Llewellyn, St Paul, MN

Eason, Cassandra, *Aura Reading*, 2000, Piatkus

Buddhism

Bechert, H. and Gombrich, R., *The World of Buddhism*, 1991, Thames and Hudson

Snelling, John, *The Buddhist Handbook*, 1992, Rider

Candles

Buckland, Ray, *Practical Candleburning Rituals*, 1982, Llewellyn, St Paul, MN

Eason, Cassandra, *Candle Power*, 1999, Blandford

Crystals and crystal healing

Bravo, Brett, Crystal Healing Secrets, 1988, Warner Books Inc, New York

Eason, Cassandra, Crystals Talk to the Woman Within, 2000, Foulsham

Eason, Cassandra, Crystal Healing, 2001, Quantum

Galde, Phyllis, Crystal Healing, The Next Step, 1991, Llewellyn, St Paul, MN

Devas and fairies

Bloom, William, Working with Angels, Fairies and Nature Spirits, 1998, Piatkus

Eason, Cassandra, A Complete Guide to Fairies and Magical Beings, 2001, Piatkus

Earth energies and sacred geometry

Eason, Cassandra, Pendulum Dowsing, 2000, Piatkus

Lemesurier, Peter, Gods of the Dawn: The Message of the Pyramids and the True Stargate Mystery, 1998, Thorsons

Martineau, John, Mazes and Labyrinths, 1996, Wooden Books

Molyneaux, Brian Leigh, The Sacred Earth, 1991, Macmillan

Sullivan, Danny, Ley Lines, 1999, Piatkus

Herbs, oils and incenses

Culpepper, N., Culpepper's Colour Herbal, 1983, Foulsham

Cunningham, Scott, Encyclopedia of Magical Herbs, 1987, Llewellyn, St Paul, MN

Cunningham, Scott, Complete Book of Oils, Incenses and Brews, 1991, Llewellyn, St Paul, MN

Price, Shirley, Practical Aromatherapy, 1996, Thorsons

Shamanism

Johnson, Buffie, Lady of the Beasts, Ancient Images of the Goddess and her Sacred Animals, 1988, Harper and Row, San Francisco

Johnson, Kenneth, North Star Road, 1996, Llewellyn, St Paul, MN

Wahoo, Dhyani, Voices of our Ancestors, 1987, Shambhala

Smudging

Alexander, Jane, Smudging and Blessings Pack, 1998, Sterling, New York

Eason, Cassandra, Smudging and Incense Burning, 2001, Quantum

Kavasch, E. Barrie and Baar, Karen, American Indian Healing Arts: Herbs, Rituals and Remedies for Every Season of Life, 2000, Thorsons

Yoga

Selvarajin, Yesudian and Haich, Elizabeth, Yoga and Health, 1978, Unwin

Sturgess, Steven, The Yoga Book, 1997, Element

Index